WHEN CARE IS CONDITIONAL

WHEN CARE IS CONDITIONAL

Immigrants and the U.S. Safety Net

Dani Carrillo

Russell Sage Foundation • New York

The Russell Sage Foundation

Library of Congress Cataloging-in-Publication Data

Names: Carrillo, Dani, author.
Title: When care is conditional : immigrants and the U.S. safety net / Dani Carrillo.
Description: New York : Russell Sage Foundation, [2024] | Includes bibliographical references and index. | Summary: "How do people manage when they are excluded from care for themselves and their families? Drawing on eighty-five interviews with low-income, Latinx immigrants, the author explores if and how immigrants access the resources they need. The book develops the concept of conditional care to describe a safety net riddled with exclusion and exceptions based on notions of who does or does not deserve care. The chapters reveal how conditional care based on immigration policy, place, and gendered roles affects immigrants' everyday lives. Through an exploration of specific barriers, and tactics by which people gain access to services and navigate this system, the author suggests strategies by which providers and policy makers could work toward a more inclusive safety net of unconditional care"—Provided by publisher.
Identifiers: LCCN 2023021572 (print) | LCCN 2023021573 (ebook) | ISBN 9780871544742 (paperback) | ISBN 9781610448956 (ebook)
Subjects: LCSH: Immigrants—Services for—United States. | Immigrants—Medical care—United States. | Latin Americans—Services for—United States. | Latin Americans—Medical care—United States.
Classification: LCC HV4010 .C37 2024 (print) | LCC HV4010 (ebook) | DDC 362.89/9120973—dc23/eng/20230831
LC record available at https://lccn.loc.gov/2023021572
LC ebook record available at https://lccn.loc.gov/2023021573

The paper used in this publication meets the minimum requirements of American National Standard for Information Sciences—Permanence of Paper for Printed Library Materials. ANSI Z39.48-1992.

Text design by Genna Patacsil.

RUSSELL SAGE FOUNDATION
112 East 64th Street, New York, New York 10065
10 9 8 7 6 5 4 3 2 1

To my safety net—thank you for your unconditional care.

May this one day exist for everyone.

CONTENTS

ILLUSTRATIONS

FIGURES

TABLES

ABOUT THE AUTHOR

Dani Carrillo is a senior researcher and civic technologist.

ACKNOWLEDGMENTS

Publication of this book would not have been possible without Irene Bloemraad and Cybelle Fox. Their mentorship and steady advocacy to share this research with a wider audience pushed me to create a strong body of work that I am proud to share with the world. Writing this book outside of academia has not been an easy feat, and I thank its editor, Suzanne Nichols, for offering me the space and support that I needed to bring my arguments and narrative to a higher level.

To the three anonymous reviewers, your earnest and comprehensive engagement with my arguments allowed me to create a richer, more compelling, and more cohesive narrative arc. To the copyeditor, Cynthia Buck, and the production manager, Jennifer Rappaport, thank you for all your effort, patience, and careful attention to detail to bring this book to publication. Cristina Mora, your time, energy, and concrete feedback allowed me to bring my full self to this work and significantly strengthened its theoretical argument. Carolina Reid, your enthusiastic support and expert feedback as a community development scholar and practitioner shaped the rigor, accessibility, and applicability of my work.

I could not have pushed through this final revision without the careful developmental and copyediting work of Juliet Kunkel and, more importantly, her emotional support and friendship. This work is a culmination of many years of planning, fieldwork, writing, and refinement. Hung Cam Thai, your mentorship opened the doors to graduate school. Phung Su, Alex Barnard, Jason Scott, and Matt Stimpson, your peer support was critical to my staying in the graduate program. Carolyn Clark and Anne Meyers, thank you for always answering all my questions with such wisdom, patience, and grace and for making me—and so many other first-generation college and PhD students—feel included.

The Interdisciplinary Immigration Workshop provided a generative and formative space to engage with a wide range of literature and cemented long-standing collaborations and friendships; thank you to every member of that workshop for creating a safe space to share works in progress. I conducted most of my fieldwork while I was enrolled in the Graduate Fellows Program at the Institute for the Study of Societal Issues, which was led by Deborah Lustig and David Minkus. This fellowship program helped me combat much of the isolation and self-doubt that students can feel, especially in later stages of graduate school. Thank you to every single graduate fellow in my cohort, and a special shout-out to Katie Keliiaa for inviting me to join the best writing group I could ask for. Janet Shim, Stacy Torres, Tessa Nápoles, and Jeff Nicklas, the various chapters I shared with you could not have been written without your thoughtful and critical support and feedback.

Scott Allard, Elizabeth Kneebone, Alexandra Murphy, Alex Schafran, and Margaret Weir, your work on the suburbanization of poverty largely inspired my fieldwork; thank you for spearheading this literature and for offering your time and guidance as I wrestled with how to meaningfully contribute to it. Esther Cho's research on the intersectionality of race and immigration status fundamentally changed the way I think about liminal legality, and the work of Shannon Gleeson and Els de Graauw in uncovering the way immigration policy is experienced on the ground inspired me to pursue a line of research that has defined the trajectory of my professional career.

I could not have completed my fieldwork without students from the Undergraduate Research Apprenticeship Program: Diana Jauregui Inez, Joyce Raya, Guadalupe Barron Vargas, Tobias Vasquez, and Celina Maiorano. Thank you, Celina, for your thought partnership and extended support for this project. Maria "Lupita" Romo-Gonzalez, I could not have published this book without you; thank you for all your support in doing research and editing multiple revisions of the manuscript.

I thank taranamol kaur, Francesca Costa, and Eric Gianella for introducing me to Code for America's work. Your commitment to justice and equity fueled my desire to join the organization, and I have experienced tremendous personal and professional growth over the past two years through being part of this work. To the entire qualitative research team at Code for America, thank you for offering a safe and energizing space to grow together in our research practice.

A special thank-you to Jazmyn Latimer, Joselyn Maser, Anu Murthy, and Kerry Rodden for helping me navigate the steep learning curve of the civic tech sector, and to Sharon Bautista for her continued support and mentorship. A special shout-out to Filsan Abikar, Kelly Benton, Camara Cooper, Ryan Hatch, Laura Maldonado, and Atzay Perez Estrada for creating and fostering safe spaces to grow and learn from and with each other. Deirdre Hirschtritt, Danny Mintz, Dustin Palmer, and Renato Rocha, thank you for offering feedback on the policy-focused portions of this manuscript.

Lindsay Bayham and Elizabeth Ohito, your friendship and thought partnership nourish me and inspire me to become a stronger researcher and advocate. Adriana Ramirez and Antonia Mardones Marshall, gracias por todo su apoyo y amistad. Writing and thinking alongside you is simultaneously energizing and healing, and I am honored to have you in my life. Erica and Katy Pool, your joy and passion for writing and storytelling brought me much levity and inspiration at just the right time. Thom Goff, I am so appreciative of our nerd sessions and the maps for this book.

To my long-standing friends, ultimate teammates, and climbing buddies, thank you for creating community, helping me stay grounded, and reminding me to take care of myself. To my family, mom, abuela, sister, and sibling—thank you for all your sacrifices, love, patience, and steadfast support for all my endeavors. Thank you for teaching me and reminding me how to be present, stay humble, embrace moments of lightness, and work toward a better world. Matthew Torres, you bring more joy to my life than you can imagine; thank you for being a thoughtful, kind, creative, and energizing thought partner, for making beautiful music, and for guiding me and so many others in reimagining an equitable and healing place for ourselves and others.

I am immensely grateful to all those who took time out of their busy lives to talk to me about their work, their struggles, and their joys in migrating to a new country. I hope this book honors all of your contributions to our world. To every person who is on the ground building and advocating for community power, gracias. Mil, mil, gracias. You are laying the foundation for generational change.

Introduction

> [It] was really difficult to [have food to] eat, to pay the rent, it was
> almost impossible. It didn't help that we didn't have access to rental
> aid. . . . [My immigration status] is a big barrier. We give the best to
> the country, but the country is not ready to give the best to us.
>
> —Pati, forty-year-old mother of three

When the COVID-19 pandemic overtook the world in the spring of 2020,
millions of Americans reeled from losing their jobs in the subsequent lock-
downs, and many from losing their loved ones to the virus as well. For the
first time in their lives, many individuals and families struggled to put food
on the table, pay their bills, and keep a roof over their heads. Some had to
swallow their pride and apply for assistance from the government in the form
of unemployment benefits, food assistance, and public medical insurance plans,
like Medicaid. These programs, which have been in existence since the 1920s,
currently provide aid to nearly 88 million people, or approximately one in
every four people in the United States.[1] In helping to keep families housed,
fed, and healthy, these assistance programs have kept people alive.

Establishing one's eligibility for these programs, however, is difficult.
A household must live at or near a poverty line based on principles established
in the 1960s, and the applicant must navigate complicated rules and paperwork to prove and maintain eligibility for services.[2] In addition, applicants
must fall within specific immigration categories to qualify for assistance. A recent
immigrant to the United States must wait five years to apply for public benefits,

and undocumented immigrants are not eligible for many programs that meet basic needs and would otherwise help them survive.[3] Policies that intentionally exclude 11 million undocumented individuals from the benefits of basic needs programs harm not only those who are undocumented but also their families— or approximately 14 million households in the United States.[4]

According to estimates from 2017, the most recent available, the undocumented population accounts for 7.6 percent of the national labor force and 9 percent of workers in California.[5] These workers pay nearly $12 billion in taxes each year.[6] Yet, despite their contributions, undocumented and Latinx[7] populations continue to be depicted as undeserving of services, as overly fertile, and as "leeches" siphoning resources from the United States.[8] The narrative that people need to deserve access to care has reinforced a historically exclusive safety net that has only become even more closed off, or conditional, for the general population over the decades and that, starting in the 1970s, was closed off to undocumented populations except in some cases of birth or near-death.[9]

How do people manage when they are excluded from care for themselves and their families? In this book, drawing on eighty-five interviews with low-income, Latinx immigrants, I explore *if* and *how* immigrants access the resources they need. Here I develop the concept of "conditional care" to describe a safety net riddled with exclusion and exceptions based on notions of who does or does not deserve care. The following chapters reveal the impact of conditional care based on immigration policy, place, and gendered roles on immigrants' everyday lives. Through an exploration of specific barriers, and tactics by which people gain access to services and navigate this system, I suggest strategies by which providers and policy makers could work toward a more inclusive safety net of unconditional care.

The forms of conditional care described in this book are strongly based on gendered roles, which shape the strategies available to immigrants for gaining limited access to the safety net. Every person interviewed for this study identified as cisgender—that is, their gender identity at the time of the interview was the same as their sex at birth (for example, designated female at birth and identified as female at the time of the interview)—and all were either a cisgender man or a cisgender woman. In using only gender binary terms ("men" and "women") throughout this book, the intention is not to deny the existence nor the importance of the experiences of transgender, agender, gender nonbinary, or intersex immigrant individuals and communities. Such erasure through omission is harmful and exclusionary and counteracts the aims of this book.[10] With this said, the next section, in relating the stories of Mari and Tomás, captures the gendered differences in strategies to access care, as well as the gendered exclusions, uncovered by this research.

A TALE OF TWO MIGRANTS

Mari was a soft-spoken woman in her midthirties whom I met in an English class at a local elementary school. While her two children attended classes, she and about eight other women gathered in the school's computer lab to learn basic English from an enthusiastic instructor. As Mari later explained to me, learning to read and write English was not an easy task because she never had the opportunity to hone her reading and writing skills in Spanish. From the age of ten, she had worked from sunrise to sunset in the fields alongside her father and brothers harvesting local crops. At the age of fifteen, she left her hometown for live-in employment in the city and visited her parents only on the weekends. By the age of twenty-five, Mari had left Mexico to join her four older brothers in the United States. She now had two sons and was a devoted homemaker in Oakland.

In her ten years of living in the States, Mari had gained considerable confidence, skills, and know-how. She had enrolled her children in programs such as the state's medical insurance program (Medi-Cal), sought food assistance through the Supplemental Nutrition Program for Women, Infants, and Children (WIC), and found services for herself and her children, such as a low-cost medical clinic for herself, a regular pediatrician for her children, and the English-language instruction offered at this school. She owed much of her knowledge to her sister-in-law, who had started helping Mari navigate the bureaucratic ropes during her first pregnancy. Even though Mari was not happy about the income restrictions and requirements for different safety net programs, she had become deeply knowledgeable about them and participated in them to keep her family healthy and fed.

Tomás's origins were not too different from Mari's. He also came from a large family in Mexico and was forced to work from a young age. His mother, whose husband had left her to raise seven children on her own, was an intimidating figure who seldom provided love and affection to her family. She told her children that nothing would ever be handed to them in life and they would have to fight for themselves. Faced with stress and abuse at home, Tomás left the family as a teenager to work on his own, taking on whatever odd jobs he could find in the city, from window washing to shoe polishing and selling trinkets. He subsisted on the 100 pesos a month he earned in these jobs—or less than $1 a day.

Tired of this unsustainable lifestyle, Tomás took it upon himself to save enough money to join a group that paid a person known as a *coyote* to guide them on the rough journey north. He was originally intent on going to New York, but when he learned that destination was beyond his financial reach, he settled on northern California instead. Tomás went with an acquaintance, Victor, whom he referred to as *"el señor."* When they arrived, Victor offered him a place to stay with his brother for the first two months until he found his own place to live. Victor and his brother directed Tomás to the different street corners where he could wait for work as a day laborer. For the first few years, he claimed, he found employment every day by standing at a corner near a local pharmacy. Tomás described this period as "the good old days," a time when he was able to save up money and not worry too much about the daily grind. As an undocumented immigrant, he didn't feel safe opening a bank account, so he entrusted his savings to Paulo, another friend and later his roommate. Little did Tomás know that Paulo would turn against him and steal his savings. His friend's theft and betrayal sent Tomás into a downward spiral.

When Tomás's savings were stolen, his dream was shattered. Gone was his chance at owning a home or a car, or even renting an apartment. He sought help at different legal aid clinics, but the lawyers couldn't take his case because it was a civil matter. Tomás now lived and slept in a closet in his landlord's basement. He tried to secure jobs from a local day labor center, where I met him, but because he was in his fifties, he was seldom recruited for physically demanding work. He stood at street corners, waiting for anyone to come by offering work, but he was usually overlooked. The day labor center staff helped connect him to places to do free eye exams and dental checkups, but he couldn't afford to pay for glasses after his eye checkup or front the cost for the dental procedures he needed because he was uninsured. Little to no safety net was available to Tomás, whose situation was the American nightmare in stark relief.

Mari's and Tomás's stories are illustrative of the gendered access to care in the United States. Their attempts to navigate exclusions using the varied and often gendered strategies available to them led to drastically different outcomes. Mari, as a woman with children in the United States, had access to programs that were conditional on her being a mother to U.S.-born children. Tomás, as a single man with no family in the United States, had little access to any form of aid to help him make ends meet.

The metaphorical "safety net" can be envisioned as a net stretched out across four corners, ready to catch anyone who falls. Some people may be falling from a narrow tightrope, others may be leaping from one trapeze bar to another, and still others may be walking a wide plank, comforted to know a net is there just in case. Whatever people's situation, a safety net is there to catch them all. I argue in this book that the U.S. safety net does not stretch nearly far enough to catch everyone who needs it. Access to the safety net is conditional: instead of being protected by a wide net, people must strategically jump to a kind of crash pad, or series of crash pads, as they are falling to meet their needs for food assistance, shelter, or health care. More crash pads are available to some people that they can land on, while others can land on only a few, if any. People having a medical emergency have a crash pad, but people needing food assistance do not.

To extend this metaphor, we can imagine the situation that people are in before they fall. Some people who are constrained in their employment situation because of their immigration status may be walking a financial and mental tightrope as they try to support family members in their country of origin. Or they may have mental or physical health conditions associated with their migration history, experiences with discriminatory behavior, or arduous work. I argue that the conditional care available in the United States provides only a sparse set of supports (crash pads) for those who are most likely to fall: the more vulnerable some populations are as they walk a narrow financial, mental, and physical tightrope, the more conditions they must meet to access care when they fall. Even though Tomás had endured decades of physically demanding labor and grief, he was more excluded than others from medical and mental health services. Mari had managed to connect to a variety of services, but her experience would have been much different had she not had children.

Gendered roles, immigration status, and place all shape conditional access to care and affect the stability and safety of future access to care. Although services and government programs are in place that make access available to people like Mari and her children, the ease of access and eligibility for programs and services can always change as the state sustains and reproduces conditional access to care. Meanwhile, individuals, their networks, and community institutions have found ways to support themselves and each other and at times to challenge the narratives that produce and reproduce narrow, exclusionary access to services for those in need. In other words, networks and institutions help guide individuals to different crash pads. People would not need such guidance toward crash pads, however, if safety nets were in place to catch them when they fall.

PUTTING THE "WELL" BACK IN "WELFARE"

For many Americans, the word "welfare" is linked to cash-aid programs and may evoke the image of a single, Black mother. This imagery originates from U.S. political campaigns that intentionally vilified Black welfare recipients in the 1960s as undeserving of this aid.[11] The reality is that those who identify as White make up the largest percentage of participants in public benefits programs: in 2014, 43 percent of those receiving assistance from U.S. safety net programs were White (25 million people), compared to 23 percent who identified as Black or African American, 26 percent who identified as Hispanic, and 8 percent who identified as Asian, Pacific Islander, Alaskan Native, or American Indian.[12] Comparing the numbers of those who benefit or not from public aid programs distracts, however, from the larger point. Framing access to the safety net in terms of who is deserving of assistance implies that some individuals or groups are undeserving of care. This logic of conditional access to care creates a restrictive safety net that pushes out those who may be most in need. Participation in welfare programs is not a marker of "laziness," and thinking about individuals who seek public assistance in those terms blames them for being poor, rather than structures for their failure to alleviate their circumstances. Those who participate in public assistance programs are in financially difficult situations, often owing to factors beyond their control, such as historically racist policies, a changing economy, and chronic health conditions.

"Welfare" is more accurately defined as promoting and supporting the *well-being* of a population, and in other countries across the world all types of programs—only one of which is cash aid—have this mission. For this reason, I explicitly use the term "care" in this book to describe programs related to food assistance, health services, and other basic needs. These are all programs that promote the well-being, or care, of groups or individuals so that everyone can eat, tend to their health, and nourish themselves and their families.

In France, Britain, and Norway, where welfare programs are much more robust, care is provided to citizens and residents of the European Union through ample payments that include unemployment benefits, disability income, paid paternity and maternity leave, and universal health insurance.[13] Surprisingly enough, the divide between U.S. social welfare spending and that of the European and Nordic countries was not as wide during the early part of the modern welfare state, from the early 1900s through the 1950s. Welfare programs in the early twentieth century were far from inclusive, as many non-White populations were left out of them in law and in practice, but those who did benefit from them were better able to become economically mobile and to build wealth that was passed on generationally (and thus gained an advantage that contributed to present-day racial inequities). Then, from the 1960s onward, as social spending in European and Nordic countries grew, the United States decreased its welfare spending, largely in response to racialized narratives that sought to exclude Black and Brown populations from social assistance they were seen as not deserving.[14]

Conditional Access to the Safety Net

The U.S. safety net has been conditional from the start. The Social Security Act of 1935 is commonly cited as the origin of the welfare state in the United States, but in fact it was the culmination of social policies and political pressures that began forming after the Civil War. Labor unions and politicians put forth various social policy solutions to offset the economic plight that the population faced after the war. In the end, three social policies gained traction: old-age pensions to Union veterans, financial assistance to single women with children who were deemed morally "worthy" of cash aid, and workers' compensation for workers injured on the job. These policies, while noteworthy, won out against more universal social policies that would have offered old-age assistance to all individuals regardless of their veteran status, health insurance, and unemployment insurance, all of which were being passed in Britain at the time. Instead, the social policies put in place in the United States combined old age with military service, widowhood, and work injuries as conditions for eligibility that signaled moral worth and therefore deservingness.[15] Moreover, mother's pensions were racially exclusive in practice: Black and immigrant mothers faced higher scrutiny for eligibility, and in some Southern states Black mothers were rendered ineligible by law.[16]

The racially exclusionary logic of U.S. social policies was made further evident with the passage of the Social Security Act; enacted in 1935, this social insurance program excluded agricultural workers and domestic workers, most of whom were African American and Mexican.[17] Moreover, African Americans and Mexican immigrants were legally eligible for food assistance and elderly assistance during the New Deal Era in the 1930s, but they were largely discriminated against at aid offices. Furthermore, as cities with larger populations of African Americans lowered their aid distribution compared to states with larger populations of White European immigrants, the racially coded and exclusive nature of aid redistribution in the United States was solidified.[18]

Following World War II, African Americans were largely denied many of the GI Bill's provisions for veterans, including mortgage assistance and funding for higher education, and it is possible, even likely, that other veterans of color were denied this assistance as well.[19] Even those who were able to benefit from these provisions were subject to housing segregation and redlining practices that devalued their property and led to their loss of wealth over time.[20] The racially coded welfare state has contributed in many ways to the current racial wealth gap, which continues to sustain deeply embedded patterns of structural inequality.[21]

The welfare state has reinforced conformity to highly gendered roles, which intersect with race to shape conditions of perceived deservingness for assistance. Men have historically had ample government benefits through their roles as veterans or laborers, and women have historically had access to benefits through their motherhood. Meanwhile, the movement to welfare rights for mothers, just like the suffrage movement, was racially exclusionary.[22] For example, through the 1960s non-White women who were legally eligible for programs like Aid to Families with Dependent Children (AFDC) were disproportionately subjected to "midnight checks": caseworkers would come into welfare recipients' homes in the middle of the night to ensure that they were not involved with a man, who could be providing for their children.[23] Women of color also faced pervasive discrimination from caseworkers who were more punitive with Black and Latina mothers than with White mothers— a documented practice to this day.[24] In these ways, race and gender have intersected to uniquely shape experiences with access to care and continue to do so.

Much of the safety net literature, when it discusses men at all, focuses only on their role as breadwinning fathers, not as caregivers.[25] In other words, the safety net, in its language and policies, assumes the role of men as breadwinners and fathers. Indeed, research on Black custodial fathers who are single points to the challenges they face at welfare offices and with subsidized childcare programs as caseworkers raise suspicions about their caregiving role.[26] With the passage of welfare reform, the state rhetoric around fatherhood did slightly shift to take caregiving into account with the emergence of parenting programs for fathers. However, the fatherhood programs still positioned women as intermediaries between men and the state.[27] Even though the welfare state has now acknowledged the wage-earning power of women and, to some extent, the caregiving capacities of men, it still reinforces narrow gendered roles for men and women as being most appropriate. The subjection of Black women and men to more scrutiny and disciplinary treatment by the welfare state adds racial overtones to these narratives.[28] Furthermore, these gendered structures and narratives exclude queer experiences by assuming that all relationships are between men and women, thus making heterosexuality a condition to access care.[29]

Scholars have closely examined the gendered and racially exclusive nature of U.S. welfare programs, but the impact of citizenship or legal immigration status on access to the public safety net is less well understood. Only in more recent years have scholars like Cybelle Fox delved into the history of welfare access for noncitizen populations. Fox has found that, prior to the 1970s, federal law often *included* noncitizens in the U.S. welfare state, even as non-White immigrants were historically excluded in practice.[30] After the 1970s, however, the welfare state started to become more legally restrictive toward immigrant populations as the rhetoric of deservingness for access to public benefits, through either citizenship status or as determined by measures of moral worthiness, took hold. These racially tinged measures of deservingness, in part produced by the racial backlash against the civil rights movement, racialized welfare recipients, framing them as non-White or categorizing them as "other." In other words, after Black women led impactful campaigns for recognition of their right to social assistance, politicians spun their rights-based narrative into a story about "lazy" Black women who did not deserve aid from the state.[31] This rhetoric not only harmed Black and Brown mothers but also stigmatized participation in cash-aid assistance programs more generally.[32] This decrease in access to public spaces, services, and goods through the logic of "deservingness" and economic austerity manifested itself in other spaces as well, including higher education, in the 1970s.[33] In other words, the public services created prior to the civil rights movement were intended for a white "public," but when the conceived public became more racially diverse, governmental entities imposed conditions to limit access to what had been universal public goods, such as free higher education.

This book examines immigrants' navigation of this conditional access to the safety net to understand just how these policies affect individuals and families, how people navigate exclusions in order to access services, and how policymakers and providers can better understand these strategies in order to structure better access to care. I also consider the perspectives of men, whose experience is often underexamined in the welfare literature. Classic works such as Carol Stack's *All My Kin* and Kathryn Edin and Laura Lein's *Making Ends Meet* focus on single mothers as they describe the reliance of single mothers on family networks to help them stay financially afloat within a paltry welfare system.[34] Joe Soss intricately lays out what these private networks teach mothers about how to enroll in government cash-aid programs and manage the bureaucratic procedures for staying in those programs.[35] In the limited work on immigrants and the safety net, scholars have also noted that women, especially mothers, navigate certain public institutions, such as schools and hospitals, more than men do.[36] In a related vein, some work explores the pressure felt by undocumented mothers to prove that they are worthy recipients of social services.[37] Missing from this literature are the voices of the single women and men who are also in need of such services as they try to navigate these programs.

This book sheds light on how individuals of a wide range of immigration statuses navigate the public and private safety nets of the San Francisco Bay Area, with a focus on undocumented populations. I spoke to mothers, fathers, and single men, all of whom were struggling financially, about the different approaches they took to accessing services depending on their social positioning, place of residence, and immigration status. I found that while both men and women often had little choice but to seek employment in informal labor markets that provided no health insurance, no unemployment benefits, and no worker protections, women who were mothers could gain access to county and state public programs, at least temporarily. Single men, by contrast, had little access to public programs, and when they did qualify for (usually limited) services, they needed more targeted interventions to gain access to them. As men and women alike encountered discrimination, bureaucratic barriers, information barriers, and administrative burdens in navigating these programs, their physical and emotional health often suffered.

Even though I use the term "safety net" to describe the wide array of public and private assistance programs for individuals and families in need, I do not mean to imply that applying for and receiving assistance is a "safe" process in any sense of the word. Applying to state welfare feels especially unsafe to those who are undocumented or who live in mixed-status households because they often must disclose their undocumented immigration status to representatives of state institutions. With rapidly changing immigration policies and executive orders, undocumented immigrants are justifiably fearful and hesitant about disclosing their undocumented status to government representatives who might use that information against them. To account for the ever-changing landscape and inherent risk of seeking government assistance, I describe the process of applying for and receiving benefits as "conditionally safe."

Given the many ways of excluding those who are seen as undeserving of care, the psychological cost of the perceived risk, and the potential actual risk of seeking services, these benefits are limited and contingent. The safety of these spaces cannot be taken for granted, despite efforts by states, nonprofit actors, and private networks to make them as accessible as possible for those in need. Yes, immigrants may persist and garner the resources they need, but at what price?

NAVIGATING CONDITIONAL CARE
AS AN IMMIGRANT

This book focuses on the experiences of immigrants living in the San Francisco Bay Area of northern California, a place that is relatively more inclusive, to varying degrees, of immigrant populations and has a relatively more expansive safety net. Accessing public benefits in the Bay Area represents a best-case scenario, but even within this setting the respondents in this study encountered a wide array of challenges different only in degree from the challenges encountered in areas with more restrictive immigration and safety net policies. The lessons learned here about the strategies used by immigrants and organizations in the Bay Area to navigate these challenges can be applied more generally in places where immigrant and non-immigrant populations alike face stricter conditions in accessing care and where the need for such strategies is even more pressing.

To understand how immigrant populations navigated the conditions to access care in northern California, I embarked on a two-year project of interviewing individuals who had migrated from Mexico and Central America as adults and were now trying to make ends meet with a limited household income. To understand how they learned about and navigated public and private forms of social assistance in the region—if they sought assistance

Figure I.1   Map of Study Sites and Bay Area Rapid Transit Routes

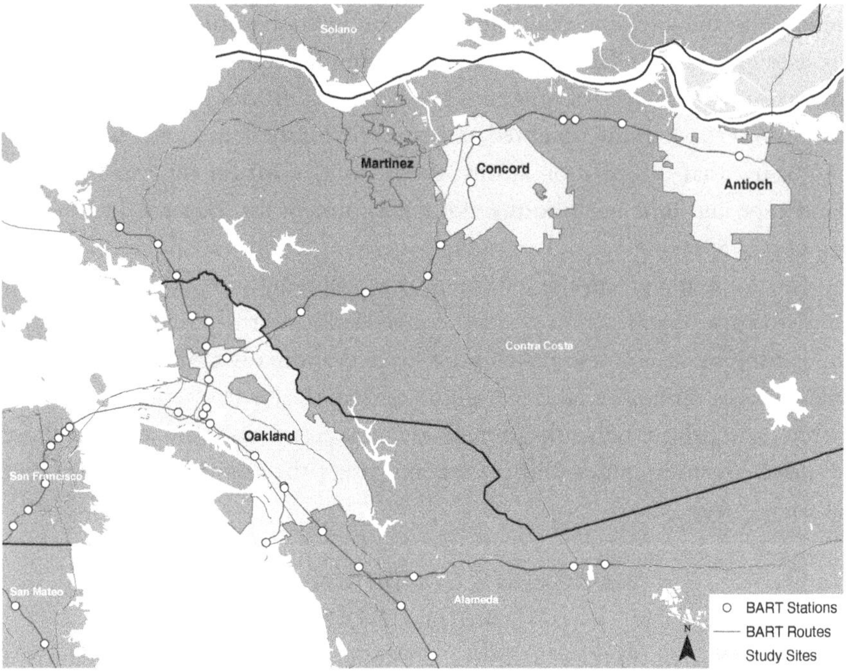

Source: Map created by Thom Goff.

at all—I started by interviewing directors and staff at several nonprofit organizations in the Bay Area. I wanted to learn who the main social service providers were in the region and how each provider viewed and conducted its work with lower-income immigrant communities. These initial interviews led to the selection of three sites for conducting participant observations and recruitment: Oakland, California (in Alameda County), and Concord and Antioch, two suburbs in eastern Contra Costa County (see figure I.1).[38]

I selected these study sites because the racial composition and the proportion of immigrants living in each community are roughly similar. Oakland is a traditional dense urban city, and more and more Latinx immigrants have moved to two of its suburbs, Concord and Antioch, where organizations taking notice of immigrants' cultural and linguistic needs have started to emerge. The demographic shifts in the Bay Area, driven predominantly by rising housing prices and acute gentrification, reflect the nationwide housing crisis and the increase in the movement of lower-income groups to the suburbs.[39] The barriers and challenges to accessing services in the Bay Area can provide generalizable insight into the conditions required to widen pipelines to aid in other sub-urban settings. The urban-suburban comparison in this project not only gave me a qualitative portrait of the impact of significant demographic changes on people's access to services in northern California but also uncovered the dynamics of similar demographic changes across the nation.[40] I address these changes in more detail in chapter 2.

UNDERSTANDING RESOURCE-SEEKING PROCESSES

In addition to the in-depth interviews, this book also draws from my expe-riences volunteering with several nonprofit organizations throughout the Bay Area that work closely with Spanish-speaking immigrant populations. I served as a Spanish interpreter at a free medical clinic and helped distribute food at churches and community-based organizations based in Oakland's eastern suburbs. I also taught English and citizenship classes at an immigrant-serving organization in Oakland, participated in Spanish-speaking prayer groups, and volunteered at citizenship workshops throughout the Bay Area.

I volunteered at these sites because I wanted to gain a better sense of the spaces where respondents went to seek material, psychological, and spiritual help and to put the interview material in the context of actual experiences and activities. However, I did not want to compromise the sanctity of private spaces, like prayer groups and medical clinics, by asking for permission to keep notes during this fieldwork, so the stories and details in this book are based only on interviews with participants who consented to the use of their interview in this research. In the methodological appendix, I discuss the research design, positionality, and methods more extensively.

While the immigrant population is ethnically and racially diverse, particu-larly in California, I focused on recruiting Latinx immigrants for interviews to limit the number of analytical comparisons in this study.[41] I recruited respon-dents through nonprofit organizations that work closely with low-income populations, including a food pantry, multiservice organizations, organizations for parents with young children, and day labor centers. I also recruited respon-dents through churches and flea markets and through other respondents. Most respondents in this sample (80 percent) grew up in Mexico; the rest came from Central American countries, including Guatemala, Honduras, Nicaragua, and El Salvador.[42] I interviewed only first-generation, adult immigrants—that is, those who were sixteen or older when they arrived in the United States. These immigrants did not grow up in a U.S. context and thus had to make the critical transition to understanding new institutions upon coming to the United States. Because I did not screen participants for documented or undocumented status, owing to the sensitive nature of this question, respondents had a wide range of immigration statuses. I also did not pre-screen participants on their income for similar reasons; instead, I asked about their income as a demographic question at the end of the interview. Because I recruited many respondents through social service organizations that catered to lower-income populations and through flea markets and churches located in lower-income neighborhoods, most respondents fit the sample characteristics. The few outliers based on income are omitted from the sample. A detailed table with demographic information on the sample and their modes of recruitment appears later in this chapter (table I.1).

For the interviews, I asked respondents about their migration history and about their experiences accessing housing, employment, and services such as health care, food assistance, education, and low-cost legal aid. Because the respondents had the most experience with food assistance and health care programs or services, those are the services I focus on in this book. I also asked about the impact of their immigration status on their day-to-day lives, including its impact on their access to food assistance, health services, and other basic needs.

I pored over the resulting data with a team of research assistants to determine the best way to code and analyze the interviews using the qualitative research software Dedoose. We used a combination of deductive coding (deducing which codes would be relevant for the interviews based on the interview guide) and inductive coding (finding codes that arose from the interviews that felt important to capture). We coded all eighty-five interviews using seven main codes and twenty-eight subcodes. The research findings in this book are based on the analysis and synthesis of these codes.

MEXICAN MIGRATION TO THE UNITED STATES: A BRIEF HISTORY

Because 80 percent of respondents in the study were Mexican immigrants, it is useful to begin by situating their biographies and migration histories in historical context. There is a long history of migration between Mexico

Table I.1   Demographic Information for Respondents in Sample

	Women	Men
N	56	29
Percentage of sample	64%	36%
Undocumented	59%	66%
Average age (years)	42	47
Average time in the United States (years)	15.5	15
Education		
Less than high school	55%	48%
High school	25%	28%
Some college/university	20%	24%
Occupation		
Construction worker/landscaper	None	14%
Day laborer	None	64%
Homemaker	52%	None
House cleaner/janitor	26%	None
Other	21%	21%
Unemployed	4%	4%
Place of residence		
Oakland	35%	60%
Concord	24%	35%
Antioch	41%	5%
Reason for coming to the United States		
To join family	57%	10%
To seek economic opportunity	37%	83%
Mode of recruitment		
Non-profit organizations	55%	66%
Church	24%	14%
Referral	8%	21%
Flea market	14%	None

Source: Carrillo 2018.

and the United States. Most of the present-day U.S. Southwest, including California, was Mexican territory prior to the late nineteenth century; even earlier this territory was—and continues to be—Indigenous land.[43] However, with the 1848 signing of the Treaty of Guadalupe Hidalgo, which ended the Mexican-American War, Mexican nationals became foreigners in their own land. Because most of them were wealthy landowners who enslaved Indigenous populations to work on their land, the Mexican population was sparse in the Southwest at the time of the treaty.[44] Migration from Mexico to the United States quickly grew in the early twentieth century, however, in response to the political revolution in Mexico and the subsequent commercialization of agricultural production. Small independent farmers were bought out by large agricultural companies to produce more and more food to meet higher demand, particularly from the United States. Additionally, newly developed train systems facilitated the ease of travel between the two countries, making it easier for Mexican laborers who were pushed out of agricultural work at home to travel north to the United States, where labor shortages made work plentiful.[45]

Several key historical moments have defined Mexican-American migration through the decades. The Bracero Program, which ran from 1942 to 1964, employed mostly Mexican male migrants for seasonal labor on farms in the United States. Immigration surged after passage of the 1965 Hart-Cellar Act, which facilitated family reunification in the United States. The 1986 Immigration Reform and Control Act (IRCA) simultaneously increased enforcement at the Mexican border and granted amnesty to immigrants already in the United States. Most recently, the North American Free Trade Agreement (NAFTA), enacted in 1994, increased south-to-north migration by incentivizing the Mexican agricultural industry to become even more commercialized; as a result, more small farmers in southern Mexico left for the United States, looking for work.[46]

The more restrictive federal immigration policies implemented in the 1990s had a great impact on migration flows. Notably, the Illegal Immigration Reform and Immigrant Responsibility Act (IIRIRA) of 1996 increased funding for border control and enforcement and toughened penalties for undocumented migrants and for those who helped individuals and groups cross into the United States without authorization.[47] This act, along with the Antiterrorism and Effective Death Penalty Act (AEDPA) passed the same year, also lowered the threshold for the felony definition to which immigrant populations were subject.[48] The pattern throughout the twentieth century was to pull in Mexican nationals to meet the country's labor demands while simultaneously pushing them out to prevent their political integration into the U.S. nation-state.

CENTRAL AMERICAN MIGRATION TO THE UNITED STATES: A BRIEF HISTORY

Apart from Mexico, respondents came mainly from two Central American countries with more recent immigration flows to the United States: Guatemala and El Salvador, which, along with Honduras, are commonly referred to as the Northern Triangle. According to a report by the Migration Policy Institute, 86 percent of Central American immigrants in 2017 came from Northern Triangle countries and comprised 8 percent of the U.S. foreign-born population.[49] As highlighted during the influx of unaccompanied minors in 2014, many Central Americans are fleeing the organized crime and gang violence that followed from the political violence of the civil wars that plagued Guatemala from 1960 to 1996 and El Salvador from 1979 to 1992. The U.S. government involved itself in the political affairs of all three Northern Triangle countries during this period by helping to fund and arm centrist parties to fight leftist rebels.[50] Even though there has been no formal civil war in Honduras, it also has experienced high levels of ongoing political instability.

In 1998, the U.S. government granted temporary protected status (TPS) to Honduran nationals following Hurricane Mitch; TPS status allowed them to live and work in the United States with a temporary, renewable permit that exempted them from deportation.[51] When two major earthquakes hit El Salvador in 2001, the United States granted TPS to Salvadoran nationals as well.

According to a 2017 Médecins Sans Frontiers (Doctors Without Borders) report, 39 percent of migrants from Northern Triangle countries reported that they had migrated north through Mexico because of "direct attacks or threats to themselves or their families, extortion, or gang-forced recruitment"; in addition, "44 percent had a relative who died due to violence in the last two years." The report also noted that 55 percent of Salvadorans reported being a victim of blackmail or extortion, and 56 percent reported having a relative who was killed in the past two years.[52] In addition to fleeing violence, most Central American migrants shoulder higher costs to make the journey to the United States, since they must cross into both Mexico and the United States, facing violence along the way.[53]

Although several Central American respondents I interviewed had been granted TPS at the time of the interview, that status was due to be suspended for Sudan, Nicaragua, Haiti, and El Salvador in 2018 and 2019. In other words, even though the U.S. Department of State had issued travel warnings for El Salvador and Honduras because of their high homicide and crime rates, the U.S. government sought to cancel the protected status of individuals who came from those countries. Guatemalan migrants have never received temporary protected status despite U.S. recognition of the high homicide rates there as well. In October 2018, after an injunction from the U.S. District Court for the Northern District of California, TPS for migrants from El Salvador and Honduras was upheld until January 2021, and at the time of this writing, that status had been extended to June 30, 2024. As long as there is no change in policy, however, TPS, as implied by its name, provides only temporary, not permanent, protection.[54]

GENDERED MIGRATION PATTERNS

With the ebbs and flows of immigration laws throughout the past century, and with an increasingly globalized economy, the gender composition of migrants has changed over the past few decades in the United States. Up until the 1960s, Mexican migrants, particularly male agricultural workers, could migrate back and forth between Mexico and the United States relatively easily. However, starting in the 1970s and intensifying in the 1990s, the U.S. government increased border control and instituted policies that punished those who came into the United States without authorization. No longer having the flexibility to return home to see those in their networks, undocumented immigrants—both longtime Mexican migrants and the increasing number of migrants from Central America—began to settle in the United States more permanently. Their settlement in the United States then facilitated the migration north of their friends, families, and hometown acquaintances.

As illustrated in the international migration literature, migration took on gendered patterns as it transitioned to a family reunification model. Previously, men had been more likely to be the first in their families to migrate to the United States, and many of them were subsequently separated—and often estranged—from their families.[55] In the 1990s, international migration became more feminized as women left their families to seek work that would economically sustain them. Unlike men, however, Mexican women migrants were more likely to have preestablished networks in the United States to facilitate their transition into the United States, even though, as Cecilia Menjívar notes of

Central American immigrants, they received limited support from these ties.[56] The migration histories of this study's respondents reflected these gendered patterns. Eighty-three percent of the men in the sample were the first in their family to migrate north, and they had weak ties, if any, upon arrival in the United States. This contrasted with the 57 percent of the women in the sample who immigrated to join their spouse or other family members in the United States. As shown throughout this book, these gendered migration patterns hold important implications for immigrants' access to social services. More detailed demographic information on respondents, broken down by gender, is shown in table I.1.

This study focuses on the stories of fifty-six women and twenty-nine men who shared many similarities. About 60 percent of respondents in the study were undocumented at the time of the interview, and 40 percent were U.S. citizens, legal permanent residents, U-visa holders, or TPS holders at the time of the interview. However, 76 percent of the total sample had been undocumented at some point in their lives. On average, respondents had lived in the United States for fifteen years and were in their forties. Most respondents had a high school education or less; 20 to 24 percent had completed some college in their country of origin. The main differences between the men and women in this study were in occupation, place of residence, and migration trajectory, and these differences were reflective of their family composition.

About half of the women in this study were homemakers; others worked as house cleaners, custodians, and entrepreneurs. Most of the men were employed as day laborers or worked in the restaurant or construction business. The geographic distribution of the women in this study was more even than it was for the men, who mostly resided in either Oakland or Concord. Finally, 57 percent of the women were primarily motivated to come to the United States to join their family, in contrast to only 10 percent of the men. Most of the men had migrated to the United States by themselves; some had left their spouse and children in their country of origin and gone north to better provide for them. As such, they had limited networks to inform them about services when they arrived in the States, as I describe in further detail later.[57]

A MOMENT IN TIME: THE ROLE OF POLITICAL TIMING IN INTERVIEWS

These interviews were carried out from the summer of 2015 through the fall of 2016, and reflect the respondents' experiences at a specific point in time when local and national policies generally seemed to be moving in a favorable direction for immigrants. People described the relief they felt from the passage of California Assembly Bill 60 (AB 60), which allowed state residents to apply for a driver's license irrespective of immigration status. The Deferred Action for Childhood Arrivals (DACA) program also made a tremendous difference in their lives, they reported, because it enabled their children to work and attend institutions of higher education. Although the 2016 presidential election came up in some interviews, the ramifications of the policies enacted after January 2017 are not captured in this research. If anything, this research was conducted during a best-case scenario for immigrants, but even then, fear of using public assistance programs was widespread. That fear only worsened with the passing of the "public charge" policy, which further deterred immigrants from applying for the public benefits for which they were eligible.[58]

The findings reported in this book on the crucial processes for accessing social services required of structurally vulnerable populations hold relevance for academics, service providers, and policymakers and can inform their outreach efforts to populations in need. By describing the exclusions experienced by migrants in a location with comparatively accessible aid and exploring how people navigate these exclusions, this book suggests strategies that could widen access even where access to assistance is relatively more conditional than it is in the Bay Area. The hope is that, with a more informed understanding of the barriers to crucial services and care as well as of the facilitators of access, institutions can better support lower-income immigrant populations.

CHAPTER LAYOUT

The following chapters uncover the multiple and overlapping barriers that Latinx immigrants may encounter in seeking access to social services. Chapter 1 provides a policy overview and detailed description of the conditional care available to immigrant populations in California. Chapter 2 focuses on the impact of placed-based conditions on access to care in suburban settings; in these contexts, immigrants face barriers to participating in programs and receiving services because of fewer organizations, smaller staffs working with fewer resources, zoning laws, and limited public transportation.

Chapters 3 and 4 detail the ways in which individuals eventually access assistance programs despite the obstacles. Chapter 3 focuses on the role of motherhood and informal coethnic networks in providing the conditions for access to care for women. As described in chapter 1, governmental programs grant temporary access to public benefits on the condition that individuals, often gendered as women, are pregnant or have young children. Having met this top-down condition for access, women are then supported by gendered coethnic networks in the United States, and they often have a "guiding figure" who helps them navigate a system of conditional care.

Chapter 4 focuses on the experience of immigrant men. The narrower set of conditions to access care that they must navigate often leads them to dismiss their need for care. These findings tie into a larger literature on the shaping of immigrant bodies for labor while also devaluing their health. Being employed serves as a condition for accessing health care in the United States, but undocumented men are excluded from the formal labor market. Within a system of conditional care, many men respond to a larger federal narrative that positively frames immigrants for their labor by embracing their identities as strong, hard workers and seek health services only in the event of a medical emergency—and sometimes not even then.

Chapter 5 focuses on immigrants' internalization of some logic of conditional care, while also contesting the logic of immigration status as a marker of morality or deservingness. In response to being criminalized and stigmatized in public discourse, immigrants emphasized their legality and strong work ethic, and sometimes they critically questioned the fairness and legitimacy of federal immigration policies and asserted their equality with others regardless of their immigration status. The counternarratives offered by immigrants at times reinforced ideas around deservingness and at other times called into question the systems that operate according to social hierarchies of who deserves to live, work, and be valued in the United States.

The concluding chapter looks toward new directions for discussions of the U.S. welfare state, especially after the COVID-19 pandemic, and sets forth proposals for socially driven, equity-focused policies. Access to basic needs, such as housing, food, and health care, is a fundamental human right and should not be limited by racial frames of deservingness. More closely examining the conditions for access built into policies, places, and institutions allows us to reimagine a more inclusive, unconditional system of care.

CHAPTER 1

Conditional Care: The Exclusion of
Vulnerable Populations from Public Benefits

Late one evening, Ramón drove to Home Depot to gather some supplies for the landscaping work ahead of him the next morning. As he loaded the materials into the back of his truck, he felt a blow to his stomach. Two men restrained him, stole all his work tools, and then took off by car. A security guard who witnessed the attack urged Ramón to call the police to file a report.

Ramón described what happened after he called 9-1-1: "The police came, and so did the ambulance. At this point, I had recently had an operation for my kidney; my main worry wasn't the assault or money. No. My main worry was that I would have complications for my kidney. . . . But I didn't want to go to the hospital because I couldn't count on my medical insurance [to cover the bill]." Like many other undocumented immigrants, Ramón was excluded from public insurance options but also barred from entering formal employment with secured benefits.[1] Under these circumstances, Ramón's access to medical care was conditional on having a medical crisis, and because he didn't know if this qualified as a crisis, he refrained from getting help when he needed it.

To understand the effort involved when patients do show up in their clinics or offices, health care providers need to be aware of the conditions they face navigating a complex social service system before they get there. This is also useful knowledge for service providers and client advocates working to streamline and improve access to services for patients in need. Individuals' interactions with social service entities, and with the bureaucrats on their staffs, have significant short- and long-term consequences for immigrant populations across generations.[2] Although the assault on Ramón did not result in complications for his kidney, other people in a similar situation may face more severe consequences from access to medical care being conditional on a medical crisis.

This chapter focuses on the various conditions that are set forth in policy and law that immigrants must understand and navigate to attempt to access care. While the previous chapter provided a brief overview of the history of conditional access to care, based on several factors, like race, gender roles, and citizenship status, this chapter provides a more detailed account of this history and focuses on the current landscape for conditional care, from the federal to the state and local levels. It also demonstrates the on-the-ground implications of conditional care for individuals in need, thus expanding the concept of conditional care to include discussions of "conditional safety" for undocumented individuals and mixed-status households. The concept of conditional safety refers to the limited psychological safety available to undocumented and mixed-status households when they attempt to participate in programs administered by governmental agencies. Faced with the ever-present threat of deportation and family separation, combined with the limiting of social services to those who qualify or are seen as "deserving" of care, individuals may feel it is too risky to seek services even when they qualify for them and even when they need them most.

CONDITIONAL CARE FOR IMMIGRANTS IN THE UNITED STATES

Before detailing the resources that are available or not to immigrant populations, it is important to contextualize the setting for restrictions in the first place. In the 1970s, a series of racialized exclusions were solidified when federal public benefits started to become legally restrictive. During this time, there was a strong conservative backlash against the successes of the civil rights movement. Feeling threatened by the calls to take action to achieve racial parity, some politicians and constituents doubled down on ostensibly more covert forms of institutional racism, such as the "War on Drugs," which led to heightened surveillance and targeting of Black and Brown communities.[3] The racial impetus behind the War on Drugs was made clear when the Nixon tapes were aired and Nixon's chief of staff was heard to say explicitly: "The whole problem is really the blacks. The key is to devise a system that recognizes this while not appearing to."[4] Politicians, like Ronald Reagan, also started to restrict access to higher education at public institutions, which had been free up until 1970.[5] Such restrictions and policies signaled a strong push to lean into a "deservingness" model for universal public goods and services, which continues to have a negative impact to this day. This impact is negative for everyone, not just low-income households. A case in point for this is student loans.

Politicians also passed a series of measures to limit the rights of undocumented individuals to access governmental assistance for basic services. From 1972 to 1976, under Presidents Richard Nixon and Gerald Ford, undocumented immigrants were excluded from Supplemental Security Income (SSI), Social Security benefits, Medicaid insurance, Aid to Families with Dependent Children (AFDC, now Temporary Assistance for Needy Families, or TANF), the Supplemental Nutrition Assistance Program (SNAP, or food stamps), and unemployment benefits—all programs from which they continue to be excluded to this day.[6]

In 1994, California voters overwhelmingly cast ballots in favor of Proposition 187 (60 percent of the vote), which would have barred undocumented immigrants from attending K-12 schools and from receiving public nonemergency medical care and social services. Moreover, it would have required social service providers to cooperate with immigration officials by handing over information on individuals' immigration status. Although this proposition was ultimately deemed unconstitutional, it brought the dark belly of racism and nativist sentiment in California to light.[7]

Soon after the demise of Proposition 187, the U.S. Congress passed the Personal Responsibility and Work Opportunity Reconciliation Act (PRWORA) in 1996. PRWORA focuses largely on limiting access to federal public benefits for noncitizens (including legal permanent residents, migrants, refugees, asylum-seekers, and undocumented immigrants). More specifically, a five-year waiting period to receive services was imposed on those who had recently been granted legal permanent resident status. The act also imposed work requirements and a time cap on people receiving cash assistance and sanctions (in the form of reduced or eliminated benefits) on families for not complying with the litany of rules specified by the TANF program. All these PRWORA policies punished single mothers and reinforced the model of a heterosexual, two-parent household.[8] This model, combined with the conditions, restrictions, and work requirements of these policies, structured the logic of who "deserved" benefits and who was "undeserving" and thus denied access to services to meet their basic needs. Moreover, a limit implemented in 1996 for many federal public benefit programs remains in place to this day: newly arrived immigrants with a green card continue to be required to wait five years to receive any type of support for basic services. The restrictions for non-U.S. citizen populations stemmed from the false assertion that immigrants were coming to the United States for public benefits.[9] Some studies have found a reduction in child poverty rates among U.S.-born parents and their children since PRWORA was passed.[10] Studies focused on non-U.S. citizens, however, have found that since the passage of PRWORA mixed-status families have been uninsured at higher rates and have experienced more food insecurity.[11]

STATE INTERVENTIONS

To offset some of these federally restrictive policies, some states, including California, have designated programs or funding to widen the conditions for accessing public benefits for immigrants. For instance, the Cash Assistance Program for Immigrants (CAPI) in California assists seniors and individuals with disabilities whose income would qualify them for income assistance through federal programs that exclude them because of their immigration status. Even within the less restrictive context of California, however, the provision of basic needs is not universally available. Rather, access to assistance is also conditional in California on criteria of "deservingness," such as labor productivity and ability or willingness to conform to traditional gender and family roles. Such criteria present the primary challenge for those committed to ensuring that all people can access the care they need.

In the rest of this chapter, I provide a broad overview of federal and California state public benefits—specifically, health care, food assistance, and unemployment—and detail the psychological, informational, linguistic, and administrative barriers to accessing them faced by immigrant individuals and families.

Health Care Assistance

Each public benefit related to health care has its own complicated set of rules and eligibility requirements—that is, its own conditions for access to care. For simplicity, this chapter focuses on the eligibility requirements based on immigration status for two public benefit programs: Medicaid and federally qualified health centers (FQHCs). FQHCs, a main source of health care services for uninsured or underinsured populations, are privately run entities that are in large part federally funded. Although Medicare is also an important part of the health care safety net, it excludes undocumented populations, and noncitizens must wait five years to qualify for it.[12] Because of the Medicare program's exclusive nature and the fact that none of the respondents discussed their experiences with it, I do not go into its policy details here.

Medicaid   Medicaid is the federal and state government-run health coverage program for adults who make 133 percent of the federal poverty line (FPL) or less. As of March 2022, approximately 81 million individuals were enrolled in Medicaid—or approximately one-quarter of the U.S. population. Overall enrollment in Medicaid and the Children's Health Insurance Program (CHIP) increased after the implementation of the 2010 Affordable Care Act, which authorized the states to increase their own income threshold to up to 138 percent. As of 2022, thirty-nine states had expanded their Medicaid programs, increasing overall enrollment in Medicaid.[13]

California's Medicaid program is Medi-Cal, the public health insurance option for many low-income Californians. Since the time of my study, access to Medi-Cal has widened. Starting in January 1, 2020, all undocumented immigrants under the age of twenty-six became eligible for full-scope Medi-Cal. Those older than twenty-six remained ineligible for Medi-Cal except in some exceptional cases: medical emergencies, pregnancies, and treatment of specific medical conditions, such as emergency dialysis for end-stage kidney disease patients.[14] In May 2022, undocumented adults ages fifty and older qualified for full-scope Medi-Cal.[15] In January 2024, full-scope Medi-Cal is expected to be available to anyone who is eligible for it, regardless of immigration status.

An applicant for Medi-Cal coverage must make 138 percent or less of the federal poverty line, which is an extremely low income in the Bay Area. In 2021, 138 percent of the federal poverty line was $17,774 for a household of one and $36,156 for a household of four. To put this into context, according to American Community Survey (ACS) data, from 2017 to 2021 the median household incomes of the sites in this study were $82,244 for Antioch, $100,011 for Concord, and $85,628 for Oakland.[16] MIT researchers calculated that in 2021, the living wage for a household of one in Alameda County was $50,463, so in order to qualify for Medi-Cal, an individual had to earn approximately one-third of the living wage. (For more details, see table 1.1).[17]

Table 1.1   Overview of Medicaid and Medi-Cal

Program Description	Conditions for Access
Medicaid: Provides health care coverage to all individuals who meet the income requirements, including pregnant women, parents, seniors, and individuals with disabilities. Children of parents with Medicaid are covered under the Children's Health Insurance Program (CHIP).	*Eligibility:* Eligibility requirements based on immigration status vary widely by state. As of this writing, fifteen states do *not* offer prenatal care to pregnant individuals if they are not of "qualified immigration status."[a] *Income:* Gross monthly income must be at or below 133 percent of the federal poverty line (FPL).[b]
Medi-Cal: Full-scope Medi-Cal, the most comprehensive state version of Medicaid in California, provides coverage for: • Outpatient (ambulatory) services • Emergency services • Hospitalization • Maternity and newborn care • Mental health and substance use disorder services • Prescription drugs • Dental • Physical and occupational therapy and devices • Laboratory services • Preventive and wellness services and chronic disease management • Children's services, including oral and vision care • Vision • Community Health Worker Services • Transportation Services • Long Term Services	*Eligibility:* Medi-Cal has more than ninety eligibility categories with unique rules and requisites. *Income:* Gross monthly income must be at or below 138 percent of FPL, which was $17,774 in annual income for an individual in 2021 and $36,156 for a household of four. *Pregnancy, disability, age, and/or parental status:* (1) Pregnant persons who earn up to 138% of the FPL are eligible for full-scope Medi-Cal, regardless of immigration status. (2) Young adults ages twenty-five and younger and DACA recipients are eligible for full-scope Medi-Cal if they meet income and other requirements, regardless of immigration status. Undocumented adults ages fifty and older qualify for full-scope MediCal as of May 2022.[c] (3) Emergency Medi-Cal is available only for emergency services to persons who meet income and other requirements, regardless of immigration status.

(*Table continues on p. 28.*)

Table 1.1   (continued)

Program Description	Conditions for Access
	Immigrant populations excluded from full-scope Medi-Cal: Undocumented individuals between the ages of twenty-six and forty-nine. In January 2024, full-scope Medi-Cal is expected to be available to anyone who is eligible for it, regardless of immigration status.

Source: Broder 2023; Medicaid.gov, "Medicaid Eligibility," https://www.medicaid.gov/medicaid/eligibility/index.html; DHCS.ca.gov, "Essential Health Benefits," https://www.dhcs.ca.gov/services/medi-cal/Pages/Benefits_services.aspx; "Full Scope Medi-Cal Coverage and Affordability and Benefit Program for Low-Income Women and Newly Qualified Immigrants," https://www.dhcs.ca.gov/services/medi-cal/Pages/Affordability-and-Benefit-Program.aspx.
[a] Broder 2023.
[b] Because 5 percent of income can be ignored for income calculations at the federal level, people whose income is 138 percent of the FPL or lower can qualify for Medicaid if their state has opted into the ACA Medicaid expansion.
[c] Broder 2023.

As I detail in the following story about Jesús, even if people are earning well below a living wage and are struggling to make ends meet, they must still contend with debts incurred by a medical crisis; those debts are even more daunting and insurmountable when respondents, owing to their immigration status, do not have access to medical insurance.

Jesús was born in Guadalajara, Mexico, and was the eldest of six. His mother dedicated herself to the home while his father sold goods at outdoor markets, or *tianguis*. Jesús was able to finish secondary school, and then he worked various odd jobs in the city from the age of fifteen. After he started going out with his future wife, she became pregnant with their first and only child. His wife had a lot of family in the United States, including an older brother who insisted that they join him. Jesús didn't want to go, but he left the decision up to his wife. His wife's brother arranged a *coyote* for them to travel with, and within a few months they arrived in the United States, in 2005.

Jesús's brother-in-law set him up right away with a job at the same demolition company that he worked at. When their daughter was old enough, his wife started working the night shift, and they took turns taking care of their daughter. The job with the company was stable and paid well; Jesús even received health insurance if he was working full-time. Within a few years, however, his marriage came to an end and his father became ill in Mexico. Jesús went back to Mexico for a couple of years to take care of his father, then returned to the United States in 2010. He was able to get his old job back. Initially he stayed with his former mother-in-law, but then a friend told him that getting a trailer would be cheaper to rent. With the help of informal loans from his friends—ranging from $1,000 to $5,000—he now lived in his trailer, paying only $600 a month for the space.

About a year earlier, Jesús had felt intense pain in his stomach area. After calling his friend for advice on whether to go to the hospital or not, he decided to call an ambulance. He thought his health expenses would be partly covered by his employer, the demolition company, but they weren't. Since he was working part-time, he wasn't working enough hours to receive health insurance benefits. When I asked him what his experience in the hospital was like, he said that the social worker "asked me where I work, and I said I worked at [the demolition company]." Asked how much he made ("around two thousand a month, five hundred a week"), he was then told that he didn't qualify for Medi-Cal. "So there's my problem."

At the time of our interview in 2016, Jesús would have had to earn less than $16,400 a year to qualify for Medi-Cal as a sole-person household. Because he earned $24,000—just enough money to cover his rent, payments on his loans, and basic expenses, with some left over to pitch in for his daughter's needs—he earned $7,600 above the income threshold for Medi-Cal. And because he was also undocumented and earned close to a living wage, Jesús now had a $50,000 medical bill that he couldn't pay.

Another respondent, Israel, said that he made a conscious effort to earn less income so that he could continue qualifying for Medi-Cal. Israel was born in a small town outside of Jalisco; his father was an *obrero*, or fieldworker, while his mother was a homemaker. Even though they had humble roots, many of his siblings, including Israel, were able to complete a university education. Israel received his degree in accounting and worked for a company for eight to ten years and then worked for the revenue department, Mexico's equivalent of the IRS.

Israel had a steady job and a home with his wife and three sons. He decided to come to the United States when he was older, however, so that his sons could have a better life. Israel's wife had brothers who had all migrated to the United States some years before, and they petitioned for their sister and brother-in-law (they were married at the time) to be granted residency status. In 1999, they traveled to Oakland for the first time to visit, and Israel worked for his brother-in-law's *panaderia*, or bakery, for a few months to make some extra cash. He and his wife returned to Mexico before making the final move to the United States in 2003. They initially moved in with his brother-in-law, then to a house they were able to afford in the Central Valley. After they lost their home there during the foreclosure crisis of 2007–2008, they bought a small home in Oakland.

Israel now worked as a chauffeur, although he wanted to continue his work in accounting. At the time of our interview, he was taking English classes at a community-based organization to work toward that goal. When I asked Israel how he started to figure out health care options when he migrated to the United States, he said:

> Well, right away, I went to [an FQHC] clinic, and I sent in my application for Medi-Cal. For Medi-Cal, I started to look at the income qualifications for it. It's also been limiting for me, because if I earn a little more than I do now, I lose the right to Medi-Cal. For someone my age, it's important for me to keep in mind. If I work now, I have to do it as a volunteer, because if not, they'll take away my Medi-Cal. And insurance right now is really expensive. My brother-in-law earns more than me, and he had a problem where he had to have a shot that costs $8,000. . . . His insurance won't cover it. It's really important for his health, and he's in a really difficult dilemma. One has to investigate and figure out what one can do.

Although Israel's appearance belied his fifty-five years of age, he was acutely aware of the medical costs that may lie ahead for him. He didn't want to end up in a predicament similar to his brother-in-law's, even if avoiding it required that he and his family scrape to get by in order to stay insured. Toward the end of the interview, Israel lamented having "lost" in migrating to the United States. He ended up taking a massive pay cut, and he struggled with expressing himself as he would have liked in English. He thought that his wife and sons probably "won" from coming to the United States: his wife had been able to take courses through several colleges, and his sons had also received a college education. At the same time, however, he was not sure that they would not also have prospered in Mexico, where his brother's sons were doing well for themselves. His mixed feelings about migration mirror the feelings of many male immigrants, especially those who find themselves separated from their families.

Health Care Coverage for Pregnant People and Children   In contrast to men, the women in this study did often talk about one important health option if they met one key condition: they were expecting a child. Prenatal care in the United States for undocumented individuals varies widely, given state-level differences in policy and interpretation of federal policy. In California, birth parents have access to insurance through CHIP for their unborn child, as well as presumptive eligibility for Medicaid, regardless of immigration status.[18] As of January 2023, however, fifteen states do not provide coverage for prenatal services for pregnant people, even if they meet other eligibility requirements for it, if they do not have "qualified" immigration status.[19] As I show in chapter 3, applying to this governmental program for coverage is not simple, but immigrant networks help smooth the process a little. Moreover, it is easier to qualify for pregnancy-related coverage in California because the income limit is higher, at 213 percent of the FPL limit (see table 1.2), and there is an additional program effective as of 2015 that expanded pregnancy-related coverage to eligible pregnant persons earning up to 322 of the FPL limit. In almost every interview, women respondents mentioned Medi-Cal as a key resource during their pregnancy. However, they did have some hesitations and concerns about this coverage.

Esperanza, for example, remained wary of signing up her children for public programs. Born and raised in a big city in northern Mexico, she said that she had had a happy childhood free of financial worries. She earned her degree in business administration right after graduating from high school but had trouble finding stable employment, despite job-hunting in multiple cities. Steeped in debt and desperate for employment, she decided to try her luck in the United States. Her middle-class status enabled her to obtain a tourist visa, and she headed north to stay with a friend who had promised her a job in his company. Unfortunately, the friend was full of empty promises, but he did connect her with another acquaintance who proved to be more helpful. Throughout the next year she was employed as a cashier at a grocery store in a suburb of Oakland. She soon met her future husband there and became pregnant with their first child. Upon learning of Esperanza's pregnancy,

Table 1.2   Overview of Children's Health Insurance Program (CHIP)
and Pregnancy-Related Medi-Cal Coverage

Program Description	Conditions for Access
Children's Health Insurance Program (CHIP): A joint federal and state program for children whose families do not qualify for Medicaid because their income is too high and who cannot afford private coverage because their income is too low.	*Income limit:* Varies by state and is determined by using modified adjusted gross income (MAGI).
Pregnancy-related Medi-Cal: California's version of CHIP provides coverage exclusively for pregnancy-related and newborn care, regardless of immigration status for those who meet income requirements.	*Income limit:* Pregnant persons who earn above 138 up to 213 percent of the FPL, or $23,434 for a household of one or $56,445 for a household of four in 2021. (Pregnant persons earning up to 138 percent of the FPL eligible for full-scope Medi-Cal.)
Medi-Cal Access Program: California-specific program that provides comprehensive coverage for pregnancy-related services; children are eligible for the Medi-Cal Access Infant Program for up to two years of age.	*Income limit:* Uninsured pregnant persons who earn over 213 percent up to 322 percent of the FPL, or $41,474 for a household of one in 2021 or $85,330 for a household of four.

Source: Medicaid.gov, "Medicaid, Children's Health Insurance Program, and Basic Health Program Eligibility Levels," updated July 1, 2021, https://www.medicaid.gov/medicaid /national-medicaid-chip-program-information/medicaid-childrens-health-insurance-program -basic-health-program-eligibility-levels/index.html; DHCS.ca.gov, "Full Scope Medi-Cal Coverage and Affordability and Benefit Program for Low-Income Women and Newly Qualified Immigrants," https://www.dhcs.ca.gov/services/medi-cal/Pages/Affordability-and-Benefit -Program.aspx.

her coworkers quickly referred her to Medi-Cal and the Special Supplemental Nutrition Program for Women, Infants, and Children for services. Since then, Esperanza had used Medi-Cal and WIC for her two other children.

When I asked her if her immigration status had made her at all hesitant to seek services for her children, she responded:

> They [the clinic staff] explained to me that there was no problem—that [I could] obtain medical attention even if I wasn't here legally . . . that my information would supposedly not go to immigration. But I think it does. To be honest, I haven't researched it well, and I don't know how true it is. But when I asked for the medical service, they said it was private and wouldn't cost anything. . . . But I don't know.

Here we see that even when she was informed by clinic staff that her information would be kept confidential, Esperanza still maintained her doubts. This isn't surprising given that such information has sometimes been compromised and medical deportations take place to this day.[20] Being highly educated may also have contributed to Esperanza's skepticism toward caseworkers. Her information was being put into a system, and there was no proof or guarantee that this information would not be shared. Other women who eventually applied for public programs like Medi-Cal and WIC described their decision using words like "fear" and "risk." As discussed in chapter 2, women respondents often described their children as their primary motivation for participating in public benefits programs.

Federally Qualified Health Centers Individuals who have no access to Medi-Cal do have access to federally qualified health centers. These health care sites provide comprehensive primary care services to historically underserved areas and populations. Health centers have a long history of federal funding dating back to the 1960s; with the passing of the Omnibus Budget Reconciliation Act in 1990, FQHCs became an officially designated legal term for health centers that receive federal grant funding.[21]

By 2021, FQHCs were prominent actors in the health care safety net system, serving one in eleven people in the United States, including one in three people living in poverty, one in five rural residents, one in five uninsured people, and nearly three million seniors (ages sixty-five and older).[22] FQHCs offer a wide range of services, including preventive health services, dental services, mental

Table 1.3   Overview of Federally Qualified Health Centers (FQHCs)

Program Description	Eligibility Requirements
As safety net providers of services typically offered in an outpatient clinic, FQHCs include community health centers, migrant health centers, health centers providing health care for those who are unhoused, public housing primary care centers, and other health center programs. Outpatient health programs and facilities operated by a tribe, a tribal organization, or an urban Indian organization are also FQHCs.	To receive services on a sliding scale, gross monthly income must be at or below 200 percent of FPL, which in 2021 was $25,760 a year for an individual and $53,000 for a household of four. Service fees are set on a sliding scale.

Source: Health Resources and Services Administration website, "Health Center Program Compliance Manual: Chapter 9: Sliding Fee Discount Program," https://bphc.hrsa.gov/compliance /compliance-manual/chapter9.

health and substance abuse services, the transportation services necessary for adequate patient care, and hospital and specialty care. An FQHC must have an ongoing quality assurance program, and a majority of its governing board of directors must be former patients who received care at the center, among other requirements.[23] For more details on the program, see table 1.3.

As important as FQHCs are to the health care safety net, they are not without their complications. For example, FQHCs require that those seeking services become members, which is not a simple process, as Manuel attested. An older day laborer from Oakland, Manuel talked about his difficulty making a dentist's appointment through an FQHC: "I can't apply [for a dental appointment] because there's no appointments, or because I'm not a member. Well, how do I become a member? . . . [The staff members] don't explain that. If I had an idea of how to do it, I would have done it, because at least it helps. My teeth are falling out."

Struck by Manuel's story, I wondered how it could be that accessing services could be so difficult through a federally qualified health center, so I visited the Alameda County FQHC website to learn about the procedure: "If you are uninsured, there may be a wait at the health clinics. It may take days, weeks, or longer to complete your registration and establish membership at a clinic. After you establish membership, you may set up an appointment to be seen."[24] As a day laborer, Manuel already had to wait a long time to obtain any form of employment; also waiting in line and figuring out all the paperwork to obtain health care was too time-consuming and burdensome, and he was left feeling frustrated and confused.

Individuals with low incomes may also find it difficult to prove their residency when applying to programs because they live in crowded or informal housing. The Bay Area has a rising population of people who are unhoused or precariously housed; many low-income residents live in their cars, RVs, or tent dwellings, or they stay with friends or relatives for short periods of time.[25] In places experiencing a housing crisis, like the Bay Area, being able to show your name on a formal housing lease can prove difficult. In my own experience working as a bilingual intake volunteer at a food pantry, I observed the visible worry in people's faces when I asked for proof of income and proof of residency. I would reassure them that if they didn't have a pay stub, they could provide an approximation of their monthly earnings. If their name wasn't on a lease, they could provide a utility statement with their name and residence on it. Most clients were able to procure this information within a few weeks, but some didn't and subsequently had to be cut from services. The requirements at this privately run food pantry were not as strict as requirements at other places, like FQHCs. Although to some people providing proof of their income and residency may seem easy enough to do, such a requirement can be burdensome for undocumented and other marginalized populations. In addition, FQHCs are not only notoriously underresourced but also harder to come by in suburban and rural places, as I explain in chapter 2.

Mental Health Services   The mental health resources available to undocumented populations are even thinner than medical resources; only FQHCs and other community clinics offer an entry into mental, or behavioral, health services.[26] Nationwide, 70 percent of FQHCs provide behavioral health services, as do 72 percent in California.[27] The California Values Act (SB 54) was passed in 2017 to make public schools, courthouses, and health facilities—including county mental health facilities—accessible to anyone regardless of immigration status. As of August 2020, however, eight out of twelve county health facilities in California have not implemented safe space policies at their institution to make them more accessible to undocumented populations.[28] This is particularly concerning given the trauma that migrants may have experienced in their home country, during their migration, or at arrival in a new country that assigned them a liminal immigration status. Such trauma is reflected in Sandra's and Fernando's stories. As a word of caution, the following paragraphs contain references to sexual assault and other forms of abuse.

A fifty-three-year-old mother of four, Sandra had a difficult life from the outset. As a child growing up in a small coastal town in Mexico in the 1960s, Sandra essentially raised her nine younger siblings. Her father suffered from an illness that left him unable to work, and her mother worked long hours as a live-in nanny to financially support the twelve-person household that Sandra sustained while her mother was away. Their living situation deteriorated when a strong earthquake hit their town, leaving their small house in shambles. Sandra resented her parents for neglecting her and was eager to leave the household with her boyfriend when she was seventeen. They married and had three children. When the youngest one was diagnosed with a serious medical condition, she and her husband made the journey to the United States with their sick son to seek help.

With her husband and son, Sandra stayed in the United States with her brother for a few months, but she missed her two other children terribly. She returned to Mexico on her own to attend her eldest daughter's *quinceñera*. Shortly after her daughter's fifteenth birthday, she made a second journey to the United States, this time with a group of strangers. She was one of two women in a group of twenty-five men led by a *coyote*—a person paid to guide people across the U.S.-Mexico border. One of the men in the group sexually assaulted Sandra and attempted to rape her at the border, and the other woman was raped by other men in the group. To make matters worse, Sandra had aggressive hemorrhoids and needed medical help as soon as her husband and brother were able to retrieve her after she had crossed into the United States.

Sandra's brother knew that she could access medical care at a federally qualified health center in Oakland. The FQHC staff was able to treat her, and they also referred her to a therapy group for individuals who had undergone trauma. Participating in the group helped, but Sandra still felt isolated and out of place in the United States. In her first years, the sound of helicopters would trigger her anxiety and fear. She explained that "one arrives in a different world [upon setting foot in the United States]. If [I heard] a helicopter,

I would hide, because I thought it was *la migra* [immigration authorities]." Sandra later suffered the premature birth of another daughter, and she still felt guilty about receiving Medi-Cal assistance to cover the cost of that birth. It had been eighteen years since Sandra last saw her oldest daughter, and in that time her daughter had given birth to a child of her own, whom Sandra had yet to meet.

Fernando's life had been similar to Sandra's, though it varied in ways typical of gendered migration patterns. Fernando grew up in Chiapas among ten brothers and sisters, and he was able to finish middle school before he started working in construction. Over the next few years, he got married and had three children. Fernando was able to support his family for many years while employed in a big warehouse construction project in his town. But when that work ended, he found few other opportunities for employment. Like many of the men I interviewed, he made the painful decision in the late 1990s to leave his wife and three children behind and to journey north alone.

Like Sandra, Fernando paid *coyotes* to guide him to the United States as part of a group of mostly other men. Fernando was held captive by his *coyotes*, however, and he didn't know for how long. Apparently, he would not be released until a friend came with more money. "I kept calling my friend, and he wouldn't pick up, he wouldn't pick up. I spent two weeks, and I would do what they told me. I would sweep, I would wash dishes, there were other people there that were locked in. Suddenly, one day at one in the morning, they called my name, and they threw me in a park. I was lucky. That was another time. Now, if we don't give them anything, they hurt you."

It is difficult to know how often migrants are held in captivity by *coyotes*, since exact numbers are hard to come by. A recent study found that 42 of 1,100 individuals, or 4 percent of those who migrated to the United States using a *coyote*, were held captive by them until they either paid or worked off what the *coyote* said they owed, which was more than originally agreed upon.[29] The rate to guide people to the United States has also risen drastically over the decades—from a going rate of $1,000 to $3,000 in 2008 to over $9,000 in 2018.[30]

After he was released in the middle of nowhere, Fernando waited on Los Angeles street corners for offers of work and slept on park benches until he could find housing with other day laborers he befriended on those street corners. He said that, as a young man, his suffering was minimal, but being held against his will and having no access to safety net services upon being released from captivity must have been traumatic to some degree.

Through the years, Fernando had worked as a day laborer, with limited and unstable income. He was now fifty-one years old, and it had been decades since he had seen his family. He grew teary-eyed and talked wistfully about returning home, but he had made no clear plan to do so. Listening to Fernando, I wondered just how soon he would visit his family in Mexico, if ever. During our conversation, he never mentioned having accessed health care or gone to a mental health provider to process the trauma of being held hostage. Had he been connected to the right resources, he might have been found to be eligible for a U-visa, which provides a pathway to residency and would have allowed him to reunite with his family. He had been able to put his children through college in Mexico, but he lived on very limited means. With no steady income, he relied mostly on wages from his volatile employment in day labor. The uncertainty of his employment situation was worrisome: Fernando was growing old for such arduous work, and the physical toll of being engaged in it for years had become obvious.

As Sandra's and Fernando's stories demonstrate, migrating is traumatic. When people place their lives and well-being into the hands of paid *coyotes*, they quickly face potential trauma if those *coyotes* turn against them and subject them to emotional, physical, or sexual abuse. Migrants are also subject to abuse from drug cartels, border patrol agents, and Mexican government officials. Using a Harvard Trauma Questionnaire, researchers found that at least 82 percent of undocumented immigrants reported experiences of trauma, and 11 percent met the criteria for post-traumatic stress disorder (PTSD) at a hospital center in New York.[31] Although official statistics on abuse at the border are not available, reports from migrant shelters have cataloged thousands of cases of physical and sexual violence at the border. Such trauma has long-lasting consequences and can worsen without proper medical care. Even once individuals cross the U.S. border, their mental health continues to be at risk. Immigrants are exposed to stressors such as exploitation in the informal labor market, social isolation, discrimination and stigmatization, and the risk of being deported back to their country of origin, where many would be separated from their families or exposed to the political violence they had initially fled.

The oppressive conditions that impact people's health are commonly referred to in the public health and anthropology literature as "structural violence" or "structural vulnerability." Poverty itself, compounded by the psychological stress of the strategies required to navigate it, exacts a heavy toll on mental health.[32] Individuals' well-being is further compromised when poverty intersects with other factors, including liminal immigration status, racialized identities, or marginalization based on sexual orientation or gender identity.[33] It should come as no surprise that depressive and anxiety disorders, such as dysphoria (a profound state of unease or dissatisfaction) and anhedonia (the inability to feel pleasure), and behaviors such as poor appetite or overeating have been found to be more common among Latinx parents who entered the United States without documentation than among those who entered with documentation. In fact, undocumented Latinx parents were four times more likely to suffer from depression than those who had documents to enter the United States.[34] Studies have indicated that when undocumented status intersects with other marginalized identities or experiences, mental health worsens.[35] These statistics are troubling for many reasons, but what makes them even more alarming is that populations already at higher risk of compromised mental health are among the least likely to be able to access the services they need.

Food Assistance

In addition to health care services, some respondents mentioned food assistance as an important public benefit. Undocumented populations, however, are largely excluded from participating in programs like the Supplementary Nutrition Assistance Program. For context, in 2020, one in every five Californians described themselves as food-insecure—that is, they did not know where their next meal was coming from.[36] Controlling for other factors such as income, household size, and geographic location, food insecurity is more common among Black and Latinx populations than among Whites, and it is even more prevalent among immigrant populations, particularly undocumented populations.[37] Table 1.4 provides more details on SNAP eligibility requirements, based on income, immigration, and parental status, in the United States and in California.

The Supplemental Nutrition Assistance Program ("food stamps") is the main federal food assistance program. As seen in table 1.4, most undocumented adults are excluded from this program. Undocumented individuals can qualify for it if their family meets the income criteria, which are well below a living wage; however, many undocumented mothers are reluctant to apply for SNAP benefits on behalf of their children. This was the case for Ximena, a thirty-nine-year-old mother of three.

Table 1.4   Overview of Federal and State Food Assistance Programs

Program Description	Eligibility Requirements
Supplemental Nutrition Assistance Program (SNAP, federal): Provides food assistance to low-income individuals and families through disbursal of individual electronic benefit transfer (EBT) cards, which can be used to purchase food at most grocery stores and farmers' markets and at some restaurants.	*Income:* Gross monthly income must be at or below 130 percent of the federal poverty line for most households. In 2021, 130 percent of FPL was $16,596 in annual income for an individual and $24,068 for a household of four.
CalFresh (state): Provides food assistance to low-income individuals and families that varies by income: the maximum allotment for the 2022–2023 fiscal year was $281 per month for an individual and $939 for a household of four; the minimum allotment for a household is $23.	*Income:* Gross monthly income must be at or below 200 percent of the federal poverty line for most households. In 2021, 200 percent of FPL was $25,760 in annual income for an individual, or $2,024 per month, and $53,000 for a household of four.
California Food Assistance Program (CFAP) (state): Provides food assistance to "qualified immigrants" and LPRs who have lived in the U.S. for less than five years, but are otherwise eligible for CalFresh.	*Pregnancy, disability, age, and/or parental status:* Legal permanent residents (LPRs) who have resided in the United States for less than five years are eligible for CalFresh if they are under the age of eighteen or are receiving disability-related assistance or benefits. LPRs who have resided in the United States for less than five years and do not meet the above criteria are eligible for CFAP. *Excluded immigrant populations:* Individuals on a student, work, or tourist visa, undocumented individuals, and all DACA and most TPS recipients.

Source: California Department of Social Services (CDSS) website, "CDSS Programs, CalFresh, Eligibility and Issuance Requirements," https://www.cdss.ca.gov/inforesources/cdss-programs/calfresh/eligibility-and-issuance-requirements; U.S. Department of Agriculture Food and Nutrition Service website, "SNAP Eligibility" and "SNAP FY 2023 Cost-of-Living-Adjustments," https://www.fns.usda.gov/snap/recipient/eligibility; https://www.fns.usda.gov/snap/fy-2023-cola; GetCalFresh website, "A CalFresh Guide for Immigrants," https://www.getcalfresh.org/en/immigrants.

Ximena's two oldest children lived in Mexico, and her youngest daughter lived with her in the United States. Because her daughter was a U.S. citizen, she was eligible for the state's SNAP program, CalFresh, and Ximena could apply for those benefits on her daughter's behalf. However, despite facing food insecurity, Ximena was hesitant about applying for this assistance. Her friends and acquaintances had told her that "there are [food] stamps, but I have the fear that in the future when [my daughter] wants to work, [the government] will take away that money. . . . If there is amnesty, or there is a way to fix [papers], it would harm us." They also told her that if the government caught her misrepresenting her situation when applying for benefits, she would need to pay back the full cost of the benefits to the government— an insurmountable cost, given Ximena's income. Even though Ximena would not have been lying about her financial situation and her daughter's immigration status, she thought it best to avoid any possible complications by not applying to CalFresh at all.

Experiences like Ximena's show us that immigration status puts up not only a material barrier to accessing services but also psychological and social barriers. Even women who were legal permanent residents or U.S. citizens were hesitant to seek services. They too thought about the repercussions of seeking services for their citizenship or their spouse's citizenship. For example, Marta, a twenty-nine-year-old U.S. citizen, was hesitant to apply for CalFresh benefits owing to her husband Miguel's noncitizen status. For much of their relationship, Miguel was undocumented—a status that made for a stressful and anxiety-provoking pregnancy. "What if the police stop us and [they see] my husband has no license? I can't [financially] support myself on my own." To help assuage her constant worries, Marta drove her husband to work whenever she could before she went to work herself. After their child was born, they decided to apply for a marriage visa, and her husband received a green card. Now they both had a relatively stable immigration status. Miguel worked in construction, while Marta took on jobs through a temp agency, but they still had trouble making ends meet, since most of their income went toward rent for their one-bedroom apartment in Oakland—rent that kept going up.

When I asked Marta if she ever used food assistance programs when they were low on money, she said, "I haven't applied for food stamps. I'm scared. Maybe I have been qualified for them, but I'm scared to ask for that help." When I asked why she was scared, she responded, "I don't know. I think that maybe with time . . . my husband might have problems with that, and he just fixed his residency, and so we still feel limitations for a little bit." Marta's anxiety demonstrates why a "safety" net that could provide food security is only a conditional safety net when it requires that the applicant take on the psychological weight of risk assessment. Other women expressed a similar fear that applying for food assistance would impact their children's chances of obtaining residency or citizenship in the future. Studies have demonstrated a similar "chilling" effect on mixed-status families seeking access to health care services. U.S. citizens and legal permanent residents are eligible for these services, but they are wary of the impact on their own or their undocumented family members' chances of citizenship in the future.[38]

Respondents reported that, instead of seeking governmental food assistance, they more often received support from nongovernmental sources like churches and community-based organizations (CBOs). Ramón explained that he had difficulty meeting his basic expenses because landscaping work dries up during rainy periods. "That is precisely why I come to this [CBO]," he said. "The [CBO] gives me medical services, meals, groceries, and helps with my housing." All of the men from the day labor organization in Oakland said that part of the initial appeal of the worker center was that it offered free hot meals in the evenings after work, with no eligibility requirement. The food was available to all who needed it; there was no condition put on access, no filtering for deservingness, and no requirement that qualification for the meal be proven. Additionally, with no paperwork to fill out that might reveal their status, immigrants found it easier to go to places like churches and CBOs than it was to apply for SNAP benefits—which, again, were not even available for undocumented individuals.

Food Assistance for Pregnant People and Guardians of Young Children

Undocumented mothers of young children are excluded from SNAP benefits, but they often take advantage of another option for food assistance: the Special Supplemental Nutrition Program for Women, Infants, and Children (WIC). The name of this program uses gendered language, referring to "women" versus "pregnant people." Nonpregnant people or guardians are eligible to apply for the program on behalf of their children, but the language describing them is also gendered: "fathers or other guardians" are eligible to apply for services if a "mother is not present."[39] Because WIC's maximum income threshold is higher than that for other means-tested public benefits (185 percent of the federal poverty line compared to 130 percent), and because

Table 1.5   Overview of the Special Supplemental Nutrition Assistance
Program for Women, Infants, and Children (WIC)

Program Description	Eligibility Requirements
WIC provides nutrition education, breastfeeding support, groceries, and referrals to other community resources for pregnant persons and parents of young children. Grocery benefits are offered to pregnant persons, parents, and children in various monthly "packages";[a] the maximum allotments are: • *For those who are pregnant and those who are (mostly) breastfeeding (up to one year postpartum):* Juice (144 fluid ounces), milk (22 quarts), cereal (36 ounces), eggs (one dozen), an $11 voucher for fruits and vegetables, whole wheat bread (one pound), legumes (one pound), and peanut butter (18 ounces). • *For postpartum persons (up to six months postpartum):* Juice (96 fluid ounces), milk (16 quarts), cereal (36 ounces), eggs (one dozen), an $11 voucher for fruits and vegetables, and legumes (one pound) or peanut butter (18 ounces).	*Income:* Gross monthly income must be at or below 185 percent of the federal poverty line. In 2021, 185 percent of FPL was $23,606 for an individual, or $1,968 per month, and $48,470 for a household of four, or $4,040 per month. *Pregnancy, disability, age, and/or parental status:* Must be a pregnant person or have children under the age of five living in the United States. *Excluded immigrant populations:* Undocumented persons with no children under the age of five living in the United States.

(Table continues on p. 44.)

it distributes services to those who are eligible regardless of their immigration status, the program has a wide participant base (see table 1.5). In 2016, approximately 1.5 million individuals participated in WIC in California, which had the third-highest coverage rates in the nation among those eligible (65.6 percent), behind only Maryland and Rhode Island.[40] California's high coverage rate is due, in part, to the state's expansive outreach efforts to families.[41]

Table 1.5   (continued)

Program Description	Eligibility Requirements
• *Package for those who are fully breast-feeding* (up to one year postpartum): Juice (144 fluid ounces), milk (24 quarts), cereal (36 ounces), cheese (one pound), eggs (two dozen), an $11 voucher for fruits and vegetables, whole wheat bread (one pound), canned fish (30 ounces), legumes (one pound), and peanut butter (18 ounces). • *Package for children ages one to four:* Juice (128 fluid ounces), milk (16 quarts), cereal (36 ounces), eggs (one dozen), an $8 voucher for fruits and vegetables, whole wheat bread (two pounds), and legumes (one pound, dry or canned) or peanut butter. • *Packages for infants ages zero to eleven months (varies based on age):* Formula, infant cereal, baby food fruits and vegetables, and baby food meat in combination with other WIC packages.	

Source: U.S. Department of Agriculture Food and Nutrition Service website, "WIC Eligibility Requirements," https://www.fns.usda.gov/wic/wic-eligibility-requirements, "WIC Food Packages—Maximum Monthly Allowances," https://www.fns.usda.gov/wic/food-packages-maximum-monthly-allowances, "WIC Publication of the 2023-2024 Income Eligibility Guidelines," https://fns-prod.azureedge.us/sites/default/files/resource-files/wic-ieg-2023-24-memo.pdf #page=3.
[a] The term "packages" is in quotation marks because people do not receive physical packages. Instead, they go through a time-consuming process of finding the food they are eligible for at stores.

WIC grocery locations, which are easily identifiable through the program's purple, red, and green logo, provide essential staples like produce, milk, and other perishable foods that WIC participants can purchase with monthly vouchers. The small grocery stores' prices are generally lower than those found at other grocery stores, but their supply is limited to WIC-approved food staples.[42] Sorting through the foods at larger grocery stores, like Safeway, that individuals are permitted to purchase through WIC can be incredibly time-consuming, as there are strict limitations on approved foods or brands. For example, one brand of peanut butter might be approved only in its crunchy version, not the smooth kind, or wheat tortillas are approved but not corn tortillas. Organic and other highly nutritious foods are often not WIC-approved.[43]

Because mothers usually enroll in Medi-Cal during pregnancy, WIC and Medi-Cal usually go hand in hand; the two public benefits programs were the ones most commonly used by the women I interviewed. Among those connected to WIC by their health care provider after going to a clinic or hospital for their pregnancy was Esperanza, whom I described earlier. Esperanza recounted her experience participating in Medi-Cal and WIC:

> My coworkers were Latinas, and they knew about WIC and Medi-Cal. When I went to have my pregnancy test, I went to a clinic in Pittsburg [an FQHC], and my friend accompanied me. She offered to take me to get my pregnancy test, and she told me there would be a social worker who would tell me if I qualified for Medi-Cal. The same social worker who signed me up for Medi-Cal told me about WIC and explained that the [WIC] offices were right in front of the clinic. [The social worker told me], "You bring the proof of pregnancy and this paperwork." And that's how it went. . . . I used WIC during my pregnancy and after my baby was born.

WIC benefits, however useful, are narrowly limited along gendered lines and tied to an individual's status as a mother. Men and women without children are unable to access this nutritional assistance.

Unemployment Benefits

Because undocumented immigrants are excluded from the formal labor market, they do not qualify for unemployment benefits at either the state or federal level. Employment assistance and unemployment benefits are available to legal permanent residents, but as with other federal programs, there is a five-year waiting period before LPRs are eligible for these benefits. In theory, undocumented workers have the right to participate in unions, receive workers' compensation, and benefit from health and safety laws in the workplace, but as I discuss in more detail in chapter 4, actually exercising one's rights as a worker can be psychologically and logistically difficult, particularly for undocumented workers.

That said, some worker centers provide living wages or form cooperatives, such as for day labor, cleaning, or food service. In 2021, there were an estimated 250 worker centers nationwide, nearly double the number of worker centers in 2005, just sixteen years earlier.[44] These worker centers, like unions, center organizing and advocacy in their work, and they have made great strides in advancing economic justice.[45] However, the dependence of many day labor centers and cooperatives on nongovernmental resources can make their funding unstable and inconsistent, with impacts on the amount of resources and number of services they can provide.[46]

Other Benefits

In addition to not being eligible for employment assistance, undocumented individuals do not have access to federal programs related to housing assistance, tax credits, Social Security, and Temporary Assistance for Needy Families (TANF), also known as cash aid. The only safety net available to them is provided by privately funded entities, sometimes augmented by state funds, though private funds are much more limited in scope.

In detailing in this chapter the public benefits available to undocumented immigrants in the state of California, I have described this population's best-case-scenario. However, even given relatively fewer restrictions on care for immigrants in California, they still face restrictions and conditions based on gender roles and ability to work. When the most marginalized are filtered out by criteria of deservingness, some who would otherwise qualify for services are excluded, because of the complicated nature of the application process or because they fear the consequences of accessing programs they do not deserve, according to the national narrative. In other U.S. states, the resources available to the undocumented population are more restricted, and receiving assistance through public benefits programs is even more heavily frowned upon by the local culture. This is particularly the case in border communities, where inland border patrol checkpoints can further restrict the mobility and freedom of undocumented individuals, making their access to care even more difficult and unsafe. Accessing services is also difficult in suburban communities, which may not have as many antipoverty resources in place, particularly services for immigrant populations. The next chapter looks at respondents' experiences with accessing services in these places.

CHAPTER 2

Place-Based Access to Care

Early on in this study's fieldwork, I met a woman named Leti, whose rich, authoritative voice belied her small figure. She and I both volunteered at a suburban church near Antioch. Leti wore a patterned pink blouse, loose black slacks, sneakers, and a lanyard with an EAT RIGHT! logo on it. She was passionate about her business of making homemade cakes. During our volunteer shift, she would flip through photos of cakes in the form of cars, cartoon characters, and flowers, ranging from an elegant wedding cake to a whimsical children's birthday treat.

I exchanged numbers with Leti, and a few weeks later I drove out to the neighboring suburb of Antioch to interview her about her life. When I pulled up to the address in a quiet neighborhood, I saw a beige one-story house whose front patio had been decorated with holiday lights. Inside the living room, I spotted a Christmas tree, a large L-shaped couch, a coffee table, and a flat-screen TV. At first glance, I had the impression that Leti and her husband were not struggling economically and in fact were living the American dream.

In my interview with Leti, however, I found out that this was far from the case. Leti and her husband, Federico, rented a small room next to the kitchen from a younger Latinx couple who owned the house. They slept on a mattress on the floor, surrounded by wooden cabinets and shelves that housed all their belongings—their clothes, several discs with children's games for learning English, a Spanish-English dictionary, and several religious books, including a Bible and children's books of biblical stories. As I found out during the interview, Leti was a deeply religious person and connected with other community members through faith-based events and groups. I also learned that she and her husband were struggling to get by.

Leti had a long and complicated migration history. She first migrated to live with her brother in Chicago in the early 1980s, right after a financial crisis in Mexico put her in what seemed like insurmountable debt. Once Leti had earned enough money working as a hotel kitchen worker in Chicago to pay off her debts, she returned to Mexico for a few years to reunite with her husband and children. When Federico's medical treatment became costly, she decided to return to the United States to earn money to pay those expenses. This time, to ensure that her husband was cared for, Leti brought him with her. They went to Concord, where they lived in tight quarters with her eldest daughter, now living with her partner. Eventually, Leti and Federico found the room they were renting in their current home.

Leti had been hustling to find money and employment for years. Each of her occasional stints of formal work in restaurants and grocery stores had been cut off by e-verification checks that revealed her undocumented status. She now made ends meet by baking cakes and other food to sell, and on the side she collected recyclable goods to sell to distribution centers. Business had been slow lately, so she had been digging into her savings every month to make rent. Her husband's medical conditions—including glaucoma, dental issues, and diabetes—were severe, and so she had become the sole breadwinner for their family.

This chapter details the ways in which place-based and spatial factors become conditions that facilitate or impede access to the safety net. As I detail later, immigrants living in suburban places encounter a series of challenges when they attempt to access the safety net, including fewer nonprofit organizations and services, fewer multilingual and culturally competent staff, less visible social service organizations, and less reliable and extensive public transportation. This chapter details the challenges that people like Leti face in a suburb, where poverty is less visible, and contextualizes Leti's story amid the broader demographic changes in the suburbanization of poverty that have been occurring not only in the Bay Area but across the country.

THE SUBURBANIZATION OF POVERTY

The geography of poverty has been steadily expanding for the past three decades. Starting in the 1990s, poverty levels in the suburbs took off at the turn of the millennium and have been growing significantly ever since. In 2015, for the first time in the United States, people living poverty in the suburbs outnumbered those living in poverty in cities.[1] At the same time, migration patterns have drastically changed: more international immigrants are migrating directly to the suburbs and other new gateway destinations.[2] With increasing poverty and immigration to the suburbs, demands for social services in places with fewer resources and less infrastructure to meet this demand have grown.[3] Academics use the term "spatial mismatch" for the uneven match between the services needed and the services available in a region; spatial mismatch is even more pronounced for immigrant populations in need of culturally and linguistically competent service organizations and providers.[4] Researchers have quantitatively documented the spatial mismatch between social service organizations and individuals living in poverty in the suburbs, but less research has been devoted to understanding how low-income—and specifically immigrant—populations access and receive services in the suburbs.

For undocumented immigrants like Leti, living in the suburbs presents its own set of challenges in accessing food, health care, and legal aid. She and other suburban residents in this study had fewer organizations to turn to for assistance, had to travel longer distances to access services, and often met with language barriers in their everyday lives. Concord is connected to larger urban areas like Oakland through the Bay Area Rapid Transit (BART) subway line, but transportation within the city and surrounding areas is not as well developed, and it is difficult to traverse these suburbs without a car. Suburban service providers also face multiple challenges: their client base often greatly exceeds their operating capacity, and they face more difficulties in recruiting bilingual experts into their organizations. Despite these challenges, one potential silver lining of service provision in the suburbs is that, in a context of fewer organizations, there are more opportunities for nonprofit organizations, schools, and city officials to work together; as a consequence, a more cohesive, albeit limited, safety net for immigrant populations and service providers alike may develop.

Before delving into my respondents' narratives, I begin this chapter by situating the study's urban and suburban sites within the Bay Area.

THE SAN FRANCISCO BAY AREA

The San Francisco Bay Area comprises nine counties, with San Francisco—the city and county—being the densest and the smallest (see figure 2.1).

San Francisco is renowned for its progressive politics, vibrant arts culture, and beautiful vistas, but in the region it is also known for its hypergentrification.

Figure 2.1   The San Francisco Bay Area

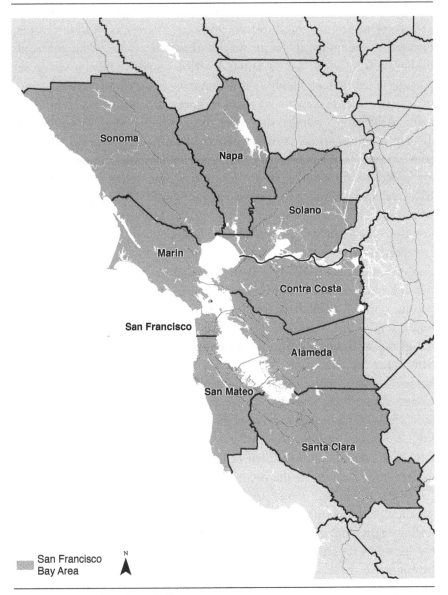

San Francisco
Bay Area

N

Source: Map created by Thom Goff.

With a median home price as high as $1 million, the city has become unaffordable for most residents of the Bay Area. The most notorious neighborhood of hypergentrification and displacement is San Francisco's Mission District, formerly a predominantly Latinx neighborhood that welcomed new arrivals in the Bay from Mexico and Central America. Extensive evictions in recent years have led to demographic shifts that have forced former residents out of the city.[5] San Francisco's northern neighbor, Marin County, is home to many of the natural wonders of the Bay Area, including Muir Woods, Mount Tamalpais, Stinson Beach, and Point Reyes. It also has highly exclusive zoning laws that restrict new housing and development, thus maintaining high prices for its ocean and mountain views.[6] Marin is not connected to the rest of the Bay Area via the BART transit system as a result of lobbying by its residents, who wanted to keep the area a restrictive enclave and make it less possible for lower-income residents of surrounding counties to commute there by public transportation.[7]

The northernmost part of the Bay Area, Sonoma, Napa, and Solano Counties, is known as the heart of California's wine country. These counties have become popular destinations for Bay Area residents seeking more affordable housing, even if they are a bit farther from the places where they have been living and working. The area is also home to vineyards and farmworkers. San Mateo and Santa Clara, the southernmost counties in the region, have become known as Silicon Valley because of the large tech companies, such as Google, Apple, Meta, and Intel, located there. These large tech companies have been a force of displacement and demographic change throughout the Bay Area, from downtown San Jose to East Palo Alto; many former residents of these areas have been priced out of their neighborhoods through gentrification.[8]

This study focused on the two eastern counties of Alameda and Contra Costa. Alameda County is nested almost squarely in the middle of the Bay Area and had a population of about 1.7 million people in 2021.[9] At the northwestern point of Alameda County is the city of Oakland, the urban site for this study; the cities of Hayward and Fremont are located to the south and Livermore to the east. North of Alameda County is Contra Costa County, where the other sites for this study are based. Contra Costa County is an expansive county with built-in inequalities. To the west is the industrial working-class city of Richmond; in the center are the more affluent suburbs of Concord, Walnut Creek, and Lafayette; and to the east are found the outer neighboring suburbs of Pittsburg and Antioch—the easternmost parts of the

Figure 2.2   The Study Sites in Alameda and Contra Costa Counties

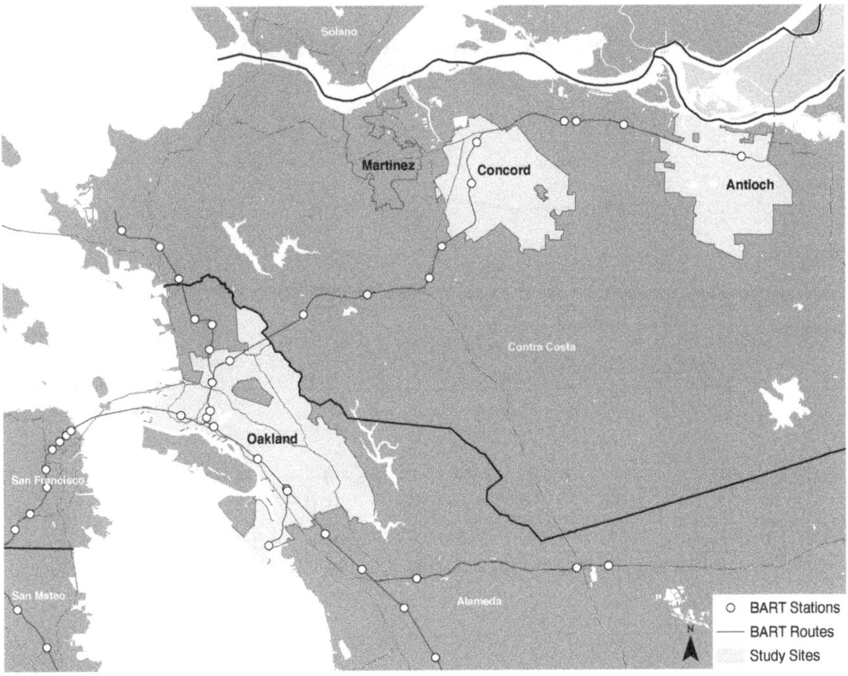

Source: Map created by Thom Goff.

nine-county Bay Area. Figure 2.2 shows the three main study sites in gray. Martinez, where respondents went to access the county's sole public safety net hospital, is highlighted in boldface.

Since the turn of the millennium, Antioch has mirrored larger national trends: the suburb's poverty levels have risen along with an influx of international migrants. While Oakland's poverty levels have remained relatively steady at around 20 percent since the 1980s, Antioch's poverty level nearly doubled in sixteen years (see figure 2.3).

Although Antioch has been featured in multiple books and *New York Times* articles about the foreclosure crisis and suburban poverty, these discussions have not included any consideration of Antioch's immigrant population—a surprising oversight given that one of every five Antioch residents is foreign-born and that number is rising.[10] In fact, the substantial and growing presence of foreign-born—and in particular, Latinx—immigrant populations is one of

Figure 2.3   Oakland, Concord, and Antioch Residents Living below
               the Poverty Line, 1970–2020

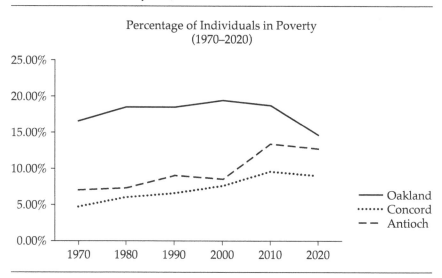

Source: Bay Area Census, n.d.-a, n.d.-b, n.d.-c; U.S. Census Bureau 2020a, 2020b, 2020c.

the common denominators of the study's sites. (See table 2.1 for demographic
information for each site.)

Oakland

The city of Oakland, home to nearly half a million residents, can make several
claims to fame: it is the birthplace of the Black Panther movement; it welcomes
refugee populations from around the world; and it has produced top athletes,
entertainment icons, and politicians, including Marshawn Lynch, Mahershala
Ali, and Kamala Harris. Oakland, like all cities, is far from monolithic. The
wealthier neighborhoods can be easily spotted in the north and far east in
the "hills," and its downtown is quickly becoming gentrified, as are the more
industrial parts of the city, West Oakland and its neighbor across Lake Merritt,
East Oakland. East Oakland is one of the most racially diverse places in the
country, and the Latinx cultural influence shines through in its bright murals
commemorating Latinx homelands and cultural roots. Many of the study's
respondents resided in East Oakland, and much of my volunteer work with
community-based organizations took place there.

Table 2.1   Oakland, Concord, and Antioch: Demographic Information

	Oakland	Concord	Antioch
Population			
Total population (2020 estimate)	440,646	125,410	115,291
Foreign-born persons (2017–2021)	28.3%	24.8%	24%
Non-U.S. citizens among foreign-born (2017–2021)	51.6%	50.7%	41.5%
Ethnic/racial composition (2020)			
Only Black or African American	22.2%	3.5%	20.2%
Only Asian	15.6%	12.5%	11.3%
Only Native Hawaiian or other Pacific Islander	.6%	.6%	.4%
Two or more races	8.4%	10.6%	11.7%
Hispanic or Latino (any race)	27.0%	29.1%	34.5%
Only White (not Hispanic or Latino)	28.5%	47.4%	27.1%
Poverty			
Persons below poverty level (2020)	14.6%	9%	12.7%
Population density			
Persons per square mile (2010)	7,004	3,996	3,611
Safety net infrastructure			
Social service nonprofit organizations (NPOs) (2022)	913	133	101
Social service NPOs with focus on ethnic/racial groups	119	2	2
Ratio of low-income population to social service NPOs	70:1	84:1	144:1
Ratio of low-income population to social service NPOs with a focus on ethnic/racial groups	540:1	5,643:1	7,321:1
Federally qualified health centers (FQHCs) (2022)	50	6	3
Ratio of low-income population to FQHCs	1,287:1	1,881:1	4,881:1

Source: U.S. Census Bureau, n.d.-a, n.d.-b, n.d.-c, n.d.-e, n.d.-f, n.d.-g; author's compilation using the Guidestar database: Candid, "Guidestar," https://www.guidestar.org/ (accessed July 16, 2022); California Department of Health Care Access and Information (HCAI), "FQHC List Public," https://funding .hcai.ca.gov/fqhc-site-search/ (accessed May 27, 2022); Healthy Alameda County 2022.
Note: The percentages for race and ethnicity in this table do not add up to one hundred because the Hispanic or Latino category overlaps with the category for two or more races.

Demographically speaking, Oakland is split in terms of racial diversity: in 2020, 28.5 percent of the population was White, 27 percent Latinx, 22.2 percent Black or African American, 15.6 percent Asian, 8.4 percent multiracial, and .6 percent Native Hawaiian or Pacific Islander. Slightly over a quarter of its population was foreign-born, and about half of the foreign-born population were noncitizens.[11] The median household income in Oakland was $80,143 in 2020, but there were vast differences across the city, from $28,114 in one neighborhood to $220,921 in another.[12] Oakland's long history of poverty and organizing is evident in the robust nonprofit infrastructure built into the city. In July of 2022, Oakland hosted 913 nonprofit organizations (NPOs)[13] offering social services such as housing, free to low-cost medical services, and food assistance; in other words, Oakland had 70 low-income residents per social service NPO.[14] In addition, the services of the Health Program of Alameda County (HealthPAC) are available to Oakland residents.[15]

Oakland has more than an average number of residents living near or below the poverty level. However, it also has an infrastructure that at least offers some support and resources to address inequalities, and its robust public transportation system, including several Bay Area Rapid Transit stops and multiple bus lines, makes it easier for residents to access different organizations.

Concord

Much less well known than Oakland, Concord lies about twenty-two miles east of Oakland. It is in the center of Contra Costa County, which is generally more affluent than the county's western and eastern regions. In contrast to Oakland, Concord has fewer claims to fame. Much of the city consists of family homes and other elements of a suburban space: expansive malls, wide, tree-lined streets, and middle-class retailers. Several downtown skyscrapers house offices and residences, and concerts for up to 12,500 people are held at Concord's pavilion. It also measures only 9 percent of its population below the poverty line compared to Oakland's 14.6 percent. At first glance, Concord seems affluent, but a deeper look reveals that a significant, mostly Latinx population lives in trailer homes and multi-unit apartment buildings in the area known as the Monument Corridor, located in the south-central part of the suburb.

Concord is less racially diverse than Oakland. In 2020, a majority of its population (47.4 percent) was White, with 29.1 percent Latinx, 12.5 percent

Asian, 10.6 percent multiracial, 3.5 percent black, and .6 percent Native Hawaiian or Pacific Islander.[16] Nearly one-quarter of its population was foreign-born, and about half of that population were noncitizens.[17] Concord had 133 social service NPOs as of July 2022, including two community-based organizations that have become staples in the Latinx community because their Spanish-speaking staff have been working for decades with the Monument Corridor community.[18] Concord has one NPO per 87 low-income residents, and the suburb has six federally qualified health centers.

Antioch

Farthest east in Contra Costa County is Antioch and its neighboring suburbs. Many readers may be unfamiliar with these suburbs, but they have become a locus of attention for scholars who follow the suburbanization of poverty because of their rising poverty levels, particularly during the foreclosure crisis. Antioch, like Concord, also has distinct neighborhoods: residential homes are located along the northern waterfront, and mixed residential spaces, including apartment complexes, are concentrated in other areas.[19] In 2020, Antioch's population was 34.5 percent Latinx, 27.1 percent White, 20.2 percent Black or African American, 11.7 percent multiracial, 11.3 percent Asian, and .4 percent Native Hawaiian or Pacific Islander.[20] As of July 2022, Antioch had 101 social service NPOs and three FQHCs.[21]

Some of the most notable differences in infrastructure among the three study sites are the health services offered. The nearest public safety net hospital for Concord and Antioch is in Martinez (see figure 2.2). Martinez is twenty miles from Antioch; accessing the hospital without a car requires a BART trip and transfer to a local bus. While Oakland has one FQHC per 1,287 residents, Antioch has one per 4,881. Of the FQHCs in Oakland, 21 offer culturally specific care, eight are school-based clinics, four specialize in mental health services, three offer dental services, and two work in conjunction with WIC.[22] By comparison, only one Concord site offers culturally specific care, and there are none in Antioch. Oakland also has 119 social service NPOs that focus on specific ethnic or racial communities, compared to only two each in Concord and Antioch. As I detail later, the limited number of organizations in Antioch and Concord, especially of any offering culturally specific services, affects service providers and clients alike.

THE DIFFICULTY OF STAFFING SUBURBAN
LEGAL AID AND MEDICAL NONPROFITS

To get a comprehensive sense of how place differences play out in the legal aid assistance sector, I interviewed directors and staff at nonprofit organizations in Oakland and the suburbs of Contra Costa County. One of this book's first interviews took place in Concord, where I spoke with John, the regional director of a legal aid NPO with multiple branches in the Bay Area, and Emily, the Board of Immigration Appeals (BIA) representative in the board's Concord branch.[23] John offered a bird's-eye view of the influence of place on the NPO's staff operations at different branches of the organization, and Emily described her experiences and struggles working as one of two full-time staff members at her organization's branch office.

When I asked about the staff capacity at the Concord branch of his organization, John lamented, "I can pretty much safely say that it's not enough. I mean, just having even a full-time attorney and a full-time BIA rep here is not enough." Being located farther away from major universities like the University of California at Berkeley and public transportation made it more difficult to fill staff positions at the organization. John explained: "It took us a while to find an attorney, even for the temporary position. It's very different; it's not like Oakland. . . . We did not have problems filling those positions [in Oakland], [but] to ask someone to come all the way out here . . . it is far away from people. . . . We're not attracting the talent coming from wherever they're living."

Because many young attorneys went to law school in places like Berkeley and San Francisco, they have already established residences there and have opportunities to work in the city where they studied. Concord and other suburbs may also not immediately stand out to prospective employees as places with high levels of need compared to Oakland, which has a longer history of poverty and immigration. Both of these factors made it difficult for John and Emily to find a staff attorney who fit their organization's needs.

Later in the interview, John and Emily spoke of having the same difficulty attracting interns to their office in Concord, in contrast to their success in hiring interns for their offices in the more urban locations of Richmond and Oakland. With fewer interns, their organizations had less capacity to take on clients, who were thus forced to wait longer to schedule appointments. I learned from interviewees who worked at legal aid NPOs in Oakland that the average wait time for an appointment was about one week. At John's and Judy's legal aid organizations in Concord, the wait time was two weeks. At the only immigration legal aid NPO branch in Antioch, the wait time was *three months.*

Pedro, the sole low-cost immigration lawyer in Antioch, was clearly over-worked. In our interview, he explained that he had personal reasons for working in Antioch: he grew up there and was more intimately aware of the need in that community. To do his job well, however, he had to wear multiple hats to keep his nonprofit organization's suburban office afloat. Pedro, who was in his early thirties, had a calm and collected demeanor as he explained his predicament:

> I'm program director for this office and staff attorney . . . because I'm the only one that can sign off on [immigration] applications. . . . I definitely don't have time to do grant and fund development, so that falls more on my supervisor . . . but it's tough, because their focus is not just funding for Antioch but the whole [regional] organization. So I think we've come to the realization that Antioch needs its specific funding as well, so I think that's what we're working on now.[24]

Pedro's office was tucked away in a commercial building accessible only by car. Perhaps because rent was more affordable in Antioch, the office was furnished with sturdy wooden furniture and framed posters that gave it an elegant feel. The organization's capacity was low, however, because only Pedro and an administrative assistant were there to hold down the fort. With just the two of them working in the branch office, it was hardly sur-prising that prospective clients had to schedule an appointment three months in advance.

A simple run of the numbers shows the massive differences in staffing and capacity by place. At the time of this study, the Oakland legal aid NPOs where I conducted interviews (including the main immigration legal aid NPOs) employed a total of fifty-two staff members and volunteers, as opposed to only six staff and no volunteers who worked at the three suburban legal aid NPOs (the main NPOs in eastern Contra Costa County) where I conducted interviews. The urban legal aid NPOs combined had well over four times the number of staff as legal aid NPOs in the eastern Contra Costa County suburbs. To put these numbers in context, according to American Community Survey estimates, Oakland was home to approximately 62,000 non-U.S. citizens in 2021, and about 25,890 non-U.S. citizens lived in Concord and Antioch.[25] Thus, while the population in need was almost 2.5 times as high in Oakland, legal aid NPOs had more than *eight times* the number of staff and volunteers to serve clients.[26]

Being understaffed impacts the quality of the services that legal aid organizations can deliver. With more staff and volunteers, more cases can be processed; moreover, a larger staff increases the number of connections between staff members and other organizations and government entities, enhancing the ability of the organization to accomplish its mission. Pedro, John, and Emily were giving it their all, but without the infrastructure and resources to scale up their services, they were always working at overcapacity, with consequences for all their potential clients in need of low-cost legal help. And when any of them became sick, their services came to a full stop.

Beyond the legal aid sector, respondents in Antioch also reported being on the phone for hours to make medical appointments at the only free clinic in the area. The clinic operated for only a few hours a couple of times a week, so those in need of medical help had to schedule an appointment only during a two-hour time slot on Wednesday afternoons. By contrast, urban residents could make an appointment on shorter notice at one of a variety of FQHCs, though, as we will see later in the book, the barrier to entry could still be high for those with limited literacy skills or specialized medical needs.

FEWER RESOURCES AND REAL ESTATE OPTIONS, MORE OBSCURE LOCATIONS

The differences in the resources of suburban and urban NPOs affect the availability and prominence of the locations that they can use for office space and thus how comfortable potential clients feel in seeking out help when they need it. Apart from two community-based organizations founded in Concord, the suburban clinics, FQHCs, and NPOs in Concord and Antioch were established as satellite offices—that is, smaller branches—of organizations based in more urban areas. Many of these spaces, besides being more difficult to access via public transportation, are unassuming and may be perceived as uninviting. Services housed in large, prominent buildings not only have greater capacity but can make newly arrived immigrants feel comfortable and welcome upon entering—as is the case at La Clínica, one of the largest FQHCs caring for Latinx populations.

La Clínica, one of the best-known FQHCs in northern California, was founded in Oakland in 1971 as a small storefront operation; over the next four decades it expanded into over forty clinics throughout the region. The Clínica location I visited in Oakland was in a predominantly Latinx neighborhood that was easily accessible via the BART system. One of eighteen Clínica locations in Oakland, this clinic provided services for over twenty-two thousand patients a year. The bright yellow building is easily identifiable: bright blue signs pointing toward La Clínica, which is walking distance from the Fruitvale BART station, show up immediately upon exiting the station. Stepping into the clinic, I immediately saw signs pointing to a variety of specialty clinics; the waiting rooms for each of these clinics were large and full. Speaking to La Clínica's large capacity and multifaceted operation was the presence of several busy receptionists at the front desk of each lobby.

In stark contrast was the suburban space in Antioch where the Clínica satellite clinic was located. Leti, the respondent discussed at the start of this chapter, learned about La Clínica from her coworkers at a grocery store she used to work at. The clinic site she visited was tucked away in a strip mall area, across from a quiet residential neighborhood in a suburb of Antioch. Established in 1999 after the nonprofit had identified a growing need for services in the area, this Clínica was one of the newer clinics. When I drove there to post flyers about this study, I had a difficult time finding it. Not only was it part of a larger building housing other businesses, but the sign for the clinic was difficult to see.

Moreover, the clinic was located in a plaza enclave that was part of a wealthy neighborhood where even I felt slightly out of place. Inside was a narrow lobby with enough seating for about fifteen people; five people waited in the lobby, including a young mom and her children. I didn't see anyone at the front desk, so I rang the bell on the counter to get the attention of a staff member. When a staff member showed up, I was taken to the back of the clinic to talk about the study in private. Only four offices were available for consults, and I could hear the soft sounds of voices coming from behind the closed doors. With the intimate layout of the clinic and the limited number of staff, getting a staff member's attention upon entering the clinic had required an extra bit of mental effort. The experience felt more socially isolated than it had in the brimming Oakland clinic.

Although a building's physical appearance seems like a minor detail, appearance can make the difference when a potential client is considering whether to step into a building or not. For example, Rosario almost didn't enter the building of one organization because she thought it was a private residence. Rosario was a young mother of three who had migrated to Antioch, where her aunt also coincidentally lived, to join her husband. After the birth of her second child, her aunt recommended that she visit a nonprofit organization that offered free parenting classes and day care for her young children. The NPO happened to be within walking distance of where she lived, so Rosario decided to visit it one day after her aunt suggested that she do that. Yet she had a hard time figuring out the exact location of the organization. She recounted:

> I told myself, "Okay, I'm going to go because I don't live too far away." So I went walking, and I couldn't find the center. As you'll notice, this place isn't like a school; it looks like a house. . . . I lost interest. Well, my aunt kept insisting . . . so one day I said, "Well, I need to find the place." I lived a bit closer this time, and I went up and down and up and down the street. And then I saw a woman with a stroller, and I asked her [in Spanish], "Hey, do you know where [the organization] is?" "Yes, it's here." "Oh God, really? No wonder I couldn't find it." Well, I came in and Lucia [a staff member] was there, and I've been going there for almost seven years.

When I first came upon the place, I was also confused. I saw what looked like a red, one-story house, but like Rosario, I couldn't see any signage to indicate that this was a nonprofit organization. Once I stepped inside, I encountered a warm and welcoming staff member who spoke Spanish, but it took a bit of extra effort to convince myself to enter the building. For immigrants seeking services, this moment of hesitation could make the difference between receiving services earlier on or not at all. Fortunately for Rosario, not only was the building close to where she lived, but once she stepped inside she felt welcomed by the staff member who greeted her.

Other immigrants seeking services, however, had to travel farther to get the care they needed, and once they arrived, entering a "safe" space such as a hospital, clinic, or school was no guarantee that they would be treated with respect, let alone communicated with in their native language. This raised the price of making a trip to seek services (both financially and psychologically) higher than was typical for urban residents. Having to travel farther increased the potential obstacles and moments of stigmatization that suburban residents might experience along the way.

THE PRICE OF MAKING THE TRIP:
THE COMPOUNDING PROBLEMS OF
DISTANCE AND LANGUAGE

The public safety net hospital for Contra Costa County is located in Martinez, which is eight miles north of Concord and twenty miles west of Antioch. Most respondents in Contra Costa County reported having come to this hospital for different kinds of medical services, ranging from emergencies to pregnancy care to other specialized services. While the hospital is not far from Concord by car, it takes much longer, over a greater distance, to get there via public transportation.

Making the trip by bus, Judy, a thirty-eight-year-old mother of three, went to the county hospital from Concord to bring her middle child to a follow-up appointment for a broken foot. On the day of the appointment, "when I arrived to register myself," she said, "I told the woman that I was there for an appointment. She asked for my name and my son's identification, but she told me that I didn't have a visit today. It was for another day, not today. I told her, 'Look, this is what the doctor gave me,' and I showed her [the] paper, because I always bring all the information with me, always."

The receptionist told Judy that she couldn't help her and suggested she go to the floor where the clinic was located to see if her son could be seen. When Judy got to the clinic, there was nobody there who spoke Spanish, and the receptionists treated her badly and started to laugh, she reported, because she didn't have an appointment and couldn't speak English. "I felt anger, powerlessness. I couldn't say anything to them because I don't know much English, to be honest." Judy and her son left without being seen.

A hospital employee in the elevator noticed that Judy was upset and asked her, in Spanish, what was wrong. When Judy recounted what had happened, the woman told her that she would help her file a report. Judy could tell her, in Spanish, what happened, and she would write it down. "I told her," Judy said,

"I came from this place . . . I came paying the bus. I also paid to have someone pick up my oldest son [from school] and to take care of him and my youngest son. So it's not fair that I am paying all of this, and then I take about an hour to get from Concord to here . . . because of all the bus stops. Who's going to pay for everything I did to come here? Who's going to pay for me coming to be told I don't have an appointment, and I have to go back?"

Fortunately, the employee was able to help Judy not only with the report but also with getting her son seen by a doctor. However, if it had not been for this employee, Judy's costly two-hour round-trip journey to the hospital would have been in vain.

Many respondents in this study, especially the women, did not have cars and either relied on personal networks for rides or used public transit. Their dependence on others for rides, combined with distance and their social isolation, could sometimes increase their risk of exploitation by their social networks.[27] As Judy's story shows, a seemingly straightforward trip can take hours in a place with limited public transportation; getting to the destination requires energy to coordinate and takes a substantial amount of valuable time that could otherwise be spent working, resting, cooking, or attending to other needs. It could also be described as a "time tax" that disproportionately affects people living in poverty.[28]

The distance between their homes and medical services mattered for many respondents; for respondents who lived in the suburbs, the distance between their home and their place of employment was also a large barrier. For example, in preparing to offer a nutrition education program for those with diabetes, the staff members and volunteers at a free clinic discussed the right time of day to hold the class and wondered what the turnout would look like. Many of those they hoped would show up spent at least an hour, if not two, commuting to their place of work, and they usually came home late. For immigrants living in the suburbs, especially for those with childcare obligations, fitting their non-work responsibilities and activities into their schedule was not easy.

Apart from the long commute times in outer-ring suburbs like Antioch, these suburbs were also farther from regional institutions like county hospitals and institutions that offered specialty care. Distance contributed to a traumatic childbirth for one respondent: she and her husband had to drive nearly forty minutes to the nearest public safety net hospital where she was scheduled to deliver her child (and where none of the medical staff spoke Spanish or relayed what was happening to her in her language in real time). Distance, combined with a weak public transportation infrastructure, was the reason it took Judy one hour and two buses to get to the nearest safety net hospital in Martinez.

Long commutes lead to significant time constraints and take a toll on sub-urban residents' health and their overall ability to seek and receive services.[29] Moreover, the effects of distance were often compounded by language bar-riers for Spanish-speaking immigrants. Judy was not the only respondent to encounter a staff unable to speak Spanish. Language barriers arose as a prom-inent theme for nearly half of the Antioch respondents, compared to only 15 percent of the Oakland respondents, and played a huge role in their access to services as well as in other aspects of their daily lives.

Leti and her husband needed to get to San Francisco for an eye surgery that Federico was scheduled to have the next day. She had been connected to La Clínica by her coworkers at a grocery store. After referring her husband to an eye specialist, La Clínica connected Leti with a local foundation in a neighboring suburb of Antioch that would cover the cost of the surgery. In preparation for the surgery, Leti and Federico had been making weekly trips to San Francisco for his appointments with the eye doctor. Each trip on public transportation took about an hour and a half each way, leaving little to no time for Leti to work that day on cooking food and cakes for income.

Two weeks after I interviewed Leti, she called me to ask for a favor. Her husband's surgery was scheduled for that week, and the foundation was covering a one-night stay at an inn in San Francisco so that he could arrive early the next morning for the surgery. Could I call the inn to confirm that they were scheduled to stay there? They had called the number, but nobody there spoke Spanish, and Leti didn't want to arrive without confirming the reservation. I agreed to make the call and was also answered by an English-only speaker who spoke harshly and quickly grew annoyed when I didn't know how to spell Leti and Federico's last name. After a few rounds of calls, I was finally able to confirm that they were scheduled to stay there. Leti breathed a sigh of relief when I let her know, and she blessed my soul.

Still, I worried about Leti and Federico making the trip to San Francisco by themselves at night and being greeted by a rude person at the front desk who didn't speak their language. I knew they would manage somehow but feared it would take a toll. I worried less when Leti told me that their daughter was going to take them to the inn, but then, the day before the surgery, Leti called me in a panic. Their daughter could no longer take them to San Francisco owing to a work conflict: Could I possibly make the trip? Doing so would cross the boundaries I had set as a researcher, but I agreed. I was already scheduled to be in Leti's area earlier that day, so I could easily drive to their place afterwards, pick them up, and bring them to San Francisco. I would be saving them at least a two-hour trip and could also translate for them when I dropped them off at the inn.

As I suspected would happen, I did need to translate at the inn's front desk. The worker there stared disapprovingly at Leti and Federico as I spoke to them in Spanish. Although I was grateful that the foundation was enabling Federico to receive the necessary surgery, I was saddened that he and Leti had to contend with discrimination and shaming during the process. Unfortunately, many immigrants are on the receiving end of such shaming every day. Many respondents, urban and suburban alike, spoke of the daily battle of feeling shamed, but the language barriers were mentioned more frequently and repeatedly in interviews with respondents who resided in the suburban sites.

For example, Pati, a forty-year-old mother of three and a devoutly religious woman, described the change she felt when she moved to Antioch from Hayward in 2010. Hayward is also a suburban area, but it is closer to Oakland and has historically been a more racially diverse suburb. She and her family had moved to Antioch after their home in Hayward was foreclosed; Antioch was the only place that offered affordable housing and had the advantage of being closer to her husband's work. Nevertheless, Pati said,

> That transition was really difficult for [my daughters] and me. I liked living in Hayward. In Antioch, everything was in English. . . . My youngest daughter didn't know English very well. There were no bilingual schools. . . . It was more difficult talking to the teachers. One feels like one is less included in the school. There were [school] meetings, but I didn't want to go because I wouldn't understand [English].

Fortunately, at the time of the interview, the school had hired a school supervisor who spoke Spanish, and bilingual interpreters became available at parent-teacher meetings. Pati now felt more comfortable and engaged in her children's education, but for three formative years she had been unable to be involved. Another parent in Antioch explained that there was no staff member at her son's middle school who spoke Spanish: "I felt like, if I needed something, they wouldn't like it very much. They didn't like that I spoke Spanish." One respondent in Concord who spoke little English said, "It affects me, because sometimes I want to talk to doctors, or people at a store, but I need to learn English, no?"

Respondents in Oakland also described the language barriers they confronted in their lives, but they spoke of how it limited their employment opportunities; no parent in Oakland mentioned language barriers coming up in their children's schools. This has important implications for parental involvement in their children's education, but also for immigrants' capacity to build more social capital and become involved in other community-based efforts.[30] A couple of respondents had sensed some discrimination when they spoke Spanish in a medical clinic, but Spanish-speaking staff were available to offer translation and interpretation support. The one notable exception was Oakland's public safety net hospital, which had—and continues to have—a limited number of Spanish-speaking medical staff.

The Suburban Silver Lining

Despite their limited resources, suburban places, even those where poverty is growing, have several advantages that can be leveraged to boost collaboration and community resources for immigrant populations. There are generally fewer nonprofit organizations in the suburbs, and they tend to be underfunded and understaffed. Suburban NPOs have responded to these constraints, however, by building strong collaborative relationships with other NPOs as well as with churches and schools to assist with outreach efforts and link clients to needed social services. Such cooperation among NPOs can streamline referral processes and produce a more cohesive set of social service providers. For example, once suburban respondents learned about one resource at a community-based organization, they could easily find out about the other NPOs in the area.

Such collaborations are particularly visible during moments of high demand, such as when Deferred Action for Childhood Arrivals was implemented in 2012. Pedro, the Antioch attorney, explained, "I think that even though there's not a lot of legal [aid] nonprofit organizations in the area, there are a lot of, more and more, each year, more nonprofit organizations in general, community-based organizations, and that's good to see. We partner a lot with a lot of these organizations just to say that we're here. We do cross-referrals as well." The other community-based organizations offer a wide range of services for low-income individuals (among whom are many Spanish-speaking immigrants) ranging from youth programs to food assistance, community organizing, and English and computer classes. The staff at the community-based organizations interviewed for this study all mentioned having referred their members and clients to nearby legal aid NPOs for immigration assistance. In fact, lawyers from legal aid NPOs held consultations in the offices of two prominent CBOs in Antioch.

The importance of NPO partnerships was reiterated by John, another legal aid provider in the suburbs: "Definitely there's a lot of partnerships, because I think we're all in the same boat. We're small offices, and as I said before, people are moving here, so the need is just continuing to grow." Bertha, a staff member at a prominent multiservice and advocacy organization, noted that a surge in demand for legal services with the implementation of DACA increased collaboration among NPOs that lasts to this day: "Right when DACA [passed], I saw the relationship strengthen with all of these nonprofits, with us to them. . . . We started getting together to see how we could work together to make sure we could get the right information to the community." In other words, NPOs came together as trusted sources of information for the immigrant community, providing resources that helped them avoid the legal scammers that sprang up in the wake of immigration reform. Community-based organizations and churches referred people to the three legal aid NPOs in eastern Contra Costa County for DACA applications. Informational workshops, or *charlas*, were held at churches and NPO offices to inform people about the DACA executive order and the application process.

In the suburbs, collaborations cut across the legal aid sector to encompass other nonprofit organizations, churches, and local government actors. When asked where he referred people and which organizations his legal aid NPO collaborated with, Pedro said, "There's First 5, there's SparkPoint . . . there's STAND for domestic violence. . . . And there's pretty big churches that we partner with. . . . So on top of community organizations, we're able to partner with churches, which we consider very important partners to get the word out." Most of the collaboration takes the form of outreach; for example, Pedro made announcements in churches about his organization's legal services and distributed organizational brochures at other organizations that offered services to low-income individuals. Pedro also worked extensively with government representatives in the agricultural community of Oakley and had close connections to the city manager, who was part of an initiative to make a growing immigrant community feel welcome in the city.

An immigration attorney at an NPO in Walnut Creek said that establishing collaborative ties across different sectors was crucial to her work. Her NPO had only begun to offer services two years earlier, so she was just beginning to get involved in the area's NPO sector. In particular, the attorney was working on outreach to Spanish-speaking clients because she spoke the language. When asked about her outreach efforts, she responded:

> Yeah, so the first year, I just tried to meet as many people as I could, to just go to meetings to meet different people, talk about my services, and then I've partnered. Now it's been a year partnered with [a day labor center in Concord] . . . so that's been great. I've also gone to Pittsburg. We used to have a staff member at [a local senior center], but he's no longer here, so I'm kind of looking for a new spot in Pittsburg, so he introduced me to many people there.

With fewer actors operating at a smaller scale in the suburbs, it was easier for this attorney to develop contacts in different organizations and build collaborative relationships.

The cooperation of legal aid NPOs with a broad range of institutions can increase the trust that low-income immigrants, and particularly undocumented immigrants, have in institutions when seeking different kinds of resources. For example, the police department in Concord, where several immigrant organizations are located, has collaborated extensively with NPOs and schools to establish trust with the low-income immigrant population. Two NPOs invite a representative from the Concord police department to come in once a week to talk to people who are victims of violence and may qualify for a U-visa. One community-based organization in Concord invites a bilingual representative from the Concord police department to meet with NPO clients twice a week to address concerns that they hesitate to bring to the police department—issues such as retrieving towed cars or reporting crime.

During my fieldwork, members of the police department regularly met with immigrant parents in an elementary school in a low-income neighborhood and asked them to share their concerns about issues affecting their communities. In Walnut Creek, an NPO staff member said that the police department "bent over backwards" to help a victim of a crime apply for a U-visa.[31] Such collaborations show the potential of building trust that allows people to turn to government entities for needed services. While it is a step forward in not having individuals go directly to the police department building for support, there could be more room for collaboration with non-policing entities who offer community-based support for reporting crimes, retrieving towed cars, or applying for U-visas. Not having to engage with the police department at all may also feel safer to many immigrants, given the documented record of abuse and racial discrimination by U.S. police departments, as most recently shown in Antioch.[32]

Collaborative relationships are not perfect, of course, and they vary between suburbs. Positive collaborations with police departments were not noted by NPOs in Antioch, for example, and other work has demonstrated that anti-immigrant sentiment in suburban areas can translate into fewer resources for immigrants and impede access to services, such as has happened in Houston.[33] That said, if the impetus is there, suburban NPOs and legal aid providers have the opportunity to work with a broader set of organizations and institutions to create a relatively cohesive institutional setting for immigrant communities. This is not to say that the more abundant resources of urban areas that enable them to offer immigrants more specialized services somehow make the spaces in which they offer those services less safe, but simply that there could be a silver lining to the relatively scarce resources available in the suburbs.

As this chapter has shown, space and place differences affect the supply of social services as well as access to them. Even as poverty in the suburbs has risen in recent years, these places still have relatively fewer organizations offering social services; in addition, the more limited transportation options in the suburbs make it harder for residents—especially those who do not have easy access to a car—to access social services. NPOs in suburban areas, particularly those that offer specialized services like legal aid, also have more difficulty attracting Spanish speakers to work at their organizations. Together, all of these factors lead to longer waiting times, fewer chances of receiving culturally informed care, and an increased risk of isolation, particularly for elderly individuals like Leti and her husband.

However, the networking mechanisms through which respondents learn about organizations and programs that can meet their basic needs remain the same across places. The following chapters discuss those mechanisms in more detail by looking at the varied experiences of immigrant men and women in accessing—or not accessing—food assistance and health care services across the sites in this study.

CHAPTER 3

"She Was the One That Moved Me": Networks and Parenthood as Conditions for Care

Rosario, whom we met earlier, grew up on the outskirts of a big city in Mexico. From the start of the interview, her sharp wit and sociable personality shone through. She had worked as a vendor in Mexico from a young age, so she was used to cajoling people and making them feel at ease. When Rosario was eighteen, she met the man who was now her husband when he was in Mexico, and after a few years she became pregnant. They decided that they would get married and that she would join him in Antioch, where he had been living for the past ten years.

Rosario did not know many people when she first arrived in the suburb but soon started forming friendships with her neighbors and her husband's friends. She became very close to one of those neighbors, Alma, who was an undocumented mother like Rosario. Alma's assistance was critical: she informed Rosario about where she could go to receive support and services, and she transported Rosario to different places, including her doctor's appointments and the grocery store. As Rosario explained:

> Not knowing English and being pregnant without knowing where to go, she was the one that moved me. She gave me rides. She said, "Don't worry. You only have to tell me when you have an appointment, and I'll take you." She took me to apply for *everything*. She took me to apply to Medi-Cal; she took me to [a place] to do my pregnancy test; she took me to [a place] to get my vitamins. If it wasn't for her, I don't know how I would have done it.

Without Alma, Rosario would have had more difficulty knowing about and accessing key services. As this book has argued, Rosario met one important, and necessary, policy condition that opened access to services for her: she became pregnant and had young children. Meeting this condition made her eligible for services, and it also increased Rosario's comfort in finding support: she was doing it for her child, not herself. However, meeting this condition was not sufficient to get access to services: Rosario's friend Alma was a crucial connecting thread for her to access services in practice. Alma could direct Rosario to the "crash pads" to cushion her fall when she experienced difficulties with access.

Like many women in this study, Rosario had a confidante, or what I term a "guiding figure"—someone who had already gone through the process of navigating conditional care. Whether they were sisters, aunts, neighbors, or coworkers, these guiding figures were vital and trusted sources of information for many like Rosario who needed help finding places to go for assistance. In seeking services they were entitled to but felt risky navigating on their own—because as an undocumented person they faced the daunting step of disclosing their immigration status—many immigrant women facing this difficulty found support in women's coethnic networks. And in turning to these networks, immigrant women became potential guiding figures themselves, in a position to open up referrals and access to resources for other women in the future. In contrast, the conditions needed to access the safety net looked much bleaker for men, as I argue in next chapter.

THE RISK OF SEEKING SOCIAL SERVICES

Seeking social services is a challenge for anyone. Even before navigating multiple agencies and submitting paperwork, individuals must take the initial step of admitting that they need assistance. Holding many of them back is the increasing stigmatization of those who seek assistance since they began to be portrayed as racialized "welfare queens" in the 1960s.[1] For undocumented individuals, seeking resources involves another important and often scary step: navigating their undocumented immigration status.

Legally, U.S. Immigration and Customs Enforcement (ICE) and U.S. Customs and Border Protection (CBP) cannot collude with public health agencies and hospitals to apprehend immigrants; nevertheless, there have been painful instances of this happening in the past.[2] The current and long-standing immigration enforcement policy of both ICE and CBP is to avoid "sensitive areas," including medical and educational institutions.[3] Despite policies providing safeguards against deportation and preserving the confidentiality of individuals' information in these spaces, however, complete safety from immigrant apprehensions or transfers to ICE or CBP is not guaranteed; moreover, these policies are subject to change depending on the current federal administration. The National Immigration Law Center, for example, advises clients not to reveal their undocumented status to medical staff if they are asked about their eligibility for public benefits, such as health insurance. Instead, they recommend stating, "I am not eligible for health insurance and do not want to apply."[4]

The National Immigration Law Center's caution is not unwarranted. As recently as September 2015, a women's health care clinic in Texas called in sheriff's deputies to arrest an undocumented woman who presented a fake driver's license to them, despite having been a patient there for eighteen months.[5] This is an extreme case of a person's "safety" being violently compromised in a health care clinic, but other cases of medical deportations have also been documented.[6] In 2013, a bill was introduced in Arizona that would have required hospital staff to call federal immigration officials or local law enforcement if individuals were not able to prove their legal residence in the United States.[7] That bill was not passed, but similar bills could be passed in the future. As with Proposition 187 in California, even though the specific legislation did not pass, the anti-immigrant sentiment motivating the bill contributed to an environment of uncertainty and fear that impacted people seeking services. The undocumented women I interviewed were well aware of the risk they took in seeking social services and described their fear of submitting their information to organizations, especially state programs. It was their children, they explained, who eventually motivated them to seek information and access to different services.

THE PRIMARY MOTIVATION FOR SEEKING SERVICES: TAKING CARE OF THE CHILDREN

Providing for her children was vital to Magdalena, a service provider and advocate at a community-based organization. Magdalena had come to the United States on a tourist visa to join her husband, who had been working construction jobs in northern California for two years. Magdalena was a preschool teacher in Mexico, but with no work permit or transferable degree in hand, she couldn't seek a job and had little to occupy her time upon arriving in the United States. After having her first child, she went into a major depression, which she slowly overcame with the help of a social worker who visited her home weekly after the birth. Magdalena then became involved with several nonprofit organizations in the area, working first as a volunteer and then serving as a board member for one of them. Now she was employed as a program coordinator.

When I asked her if her immigration status made her afraid at first to reach out to organizations, Magdalena responded, "Yes, always. I always . . . I always had fear, and I always have fear [seeking out resources]. But I say to myself, '[I do this] because I have to live, I have to do things.'" Later in the interview, Magdalena recounted a moment when she felt one of the many negative repercussions of her immigration status: she could not volunteer to drive her children's classmates on a field trip and was too ashamed to tell the teacher why: she did not have a driver's license. She said, "It's difficult, but I tell myself all the time, all the time I have to take risks, because of the strength that the kids give one, no? Of saying, they have to keep living." Indeed, all of the mothers I recruited for interviews at one nonprofit organization said that they had sought the organization's services to take care of their children. Many immigrant women first sought services at nonprofit organizations in order to meet the needs of their children. Expectant mothers, for example, had to go to hospitals for prenatal care; through the hospital, they were then able to find out about other services for their children. Even though seeking services was a scary step to take, they had decided to do it.

Maria, a single mother of two, was working hard to make ends meet living in the middle-class suburb of Concord. When I asked her if she had any hesitation or fear about disclosing her undocumented status at a hospital, she responded, "For a moment, yes. But, I think that, in moments when you know that this is your child's life . . . I think this is something that pushes you." Rosa, also a single mother of two, expressed a similar sentiment. When I asked her if she was afraid or hesitant to go to a hospital to seek prenatal care, she said that she was not. "I knew that I had to go [to the hospital] or find medical attention because this was my son's life." Rosa's concern for her children eclipsed all other problems or concerns.

Several mothers described having overcome their fear of learning to drive and driving without a license to meet the needs of their children. Some had to drive to doctor's appointments in other cities to access the only available prenatal health care for undocumented individuals, and others had to take their children to hospitals far from home to receive specialized care.

MANAGING THE FEAR OF SEEKING SERVICES FROM THE STATE: PREEMPTIVE CHECKS

The fear of seeking services was prevalent throughout the interviews with immigrant women, and many of them expressed the most anxiety about signing up for state-based programs, such as WIC or Medi-Cal. In considering whether to seek these services, respondents often conducted a preemptive check by asking friends and acquaintances if their immigration status would prevent them from seeking services or put them at risk. Over time they became more confident about asking intake workers about the paperwork and eligibility requirements for their programs.

Paloma was an extroverted forty-year-old mother of three young children. When not cooking, cleaning, and attending to other chores, she busily scurried from one child's extracurricular activity to another. She had immigrated to the United States from Mexico on a visa obtained through her husband, but when she had trouble renewing the visa, she lost her documented status in the United States. Her husband worked long hours in construction, but on rainy days or during low employment periods in the winter, it could be hard for them to make ends meet. Although she was hesitant at first, she decided to seek food assistance at a community-based organization; it was about a half-hour drive from her apartment, and she had found out about it through a friend. I asked Paloma if she had any qualms about approaching this organization because of her immigration status. At first, she replied, she was scared to seek services for her children through the county, but over time she had learned through her friends that she must simply be upfront with people about lacking a Social Security number, which would have proven she was eligible for services. "Because the first question they ask is if you are a legal resident or not. So then I told her, 'I'm not a legal resident.' . . . She told me, 'It doesn't matter. This will only cover your children.' . . . But, [now] that is always what I ask. 'Okay, what do I need to apply? I don't have a Social Security number.' That is always the first thing I say."

Paloma had reduced her fear of revealing her undocumented status by acquiring more experience in seeking support for her children. Later in our interview, she said that being upfront about not having a Social Security number also ensured that she didn't waste a staff member's time by putting them through the process of ultimately determining that she was not eligible for services. For the most part, however, she tried to avoid seeking food assistance whenever possible. She sold homemade gelatins and was paid to pick other children up from school. Like many other people I interviewed, Paloma responded to lean times by first using informal means to make extra money. Only when that did not provide enough did she seek out services.

Marisol, a custodian and forty-year-old mother of three, was also hesitant to seek assistance at first, particularly from state institutions. Her father, who had lived in the suburb of Concord for four years, directed her to a federally qualified health center when one of her children became ill. Social workers at the medical clinic asked Marisol if she was on WIC and suggested that she apply for it. She decided to do that, but not without checking her sources first. She explained that she had had no fear of seeking services at the FQHC, but that "where I did have it was at, let's say, Medi-Cal, because—because I don't have papers, what's going to happen? That's where I did hold myself back a bit, because I didn't know." But then, she reported, her friend told her, " 'There's no problem. You can go there.' So I went."

Even though both Paloma and Marisol were concerned about revealing their immigration status to state institutions, they went ahead and asked upfront about the documentation needed to receive services. This preemptive check was a protective mechanism that served to ensure that their immigration status would not be used against them when they attempted to access services. Other women who were responsible for procuring health care and childcare for their family described similar preemptive checks they made to see how their immigration status could impact their access to resources.

THE ROLE OF NETWORKS IN LEARNING WHERE TO LAND

Although twenty of the women I interviewed were documented at the time of the interview, most of them had been undocumented when they first arrived in the United States. Thus, most of them had been faced with the problem of revealing their immigration status to bureaucracies. However, even the six Latinx immigrant women who had papers coming into the country had to figure out how to access services upon arriving in the United States. They did so with the assistance of "guiding figures" and coethnic ties, and their medical conditions (often pregnancy) also facilitated their access to services.

Guiding Figures

Over half of the women in this study reported having a guiding figure who provided them with critical support in accessing important information and services. The guiding figure for most respondents was somebody who had migrated to the United States several years earlier and who shared an undocumented immigration status. For some respondents, their guiding figure was a close relative who facilitated their migration to the United States. I use the term "guiding figure" because respondents themselves described the actions of the people who helped them navigate services in the United States as "guiding" or "orienting." Instead of relying on a constellation of networks to gain information about one service or another, respondents could reliably count on one or two people to orient them to a variety of services, from local clinics to school registration to food assistance centers.

For Judy, whom we met earlier, her sister Ana served as a guiding figure. Judy had come to the United States on a whim after her older siblings who lived in the United States, including Ana, visited her and recommended that Judy and her husband make the trip north together. Ana told Judy that there was a job opening at the grocery store where she worked. Judy made the treacherous journey across the desert with her husband, and after they arrived, Ana offered Judy and her husband a place to stay while they became financially stable enough to make rent.

Ana also informed Judy about Medi-Cal, drove her to the Medi-Cal office, and helped her fill out all the needed forms. When I asked Judy if she was hesitant at first to sign up for Medi-Cal, given her immigration status, she responded: "Yes, but the big advantage was my sister . . . because my sister was there, and she already had her three children . . . she already knew a little more about how the system was, and she helped me apply. She helped me fill out the forms, bring the forms in. She taught me, and she guided me." Ana was also undocumented, so Judy knew that if her sister was able to safely apply for benefits, she would be able to as well. The narratives of many other respondents were similar; they became more confident about seeking services when they received information on those services from somebody who was also undocumented.

Another guiding figure in Judy's life was her friend, now *comadre* (her son's godparent), who told her about receiving food assistance through a multiservice center. Judy recounted, "I knew about [the multiservice organization] through my *comadre*. . . . She noticed the needs that I had . . . so she told me, 'Look, come with me, I go ask for food at [the organization], and I also go to two churches.'" Together they went to seek food assistance when needed. Her friend also told her about an NPO that would provide early schooling and day care for her young children; Judy was able to take English classes there as well.

Other respondents had neighbors, sisters-in-law, a church, or hometown acquaintances who oriented them toward social services in the United States. Who that person was and the amount of support they could provide largely depended on their immigration history (for example, whether they came to the United States to reunite with a family member or came alone). Rosario, for example, received the most support from her neighbor Alma. Her husband provided her with emotional support and a place to stay, of course, but his knowledge of social services in the area was limited. Rosario had to reach out to neighbors to find out what was available for her and her U.S.-born children, and Alma was happy to step in and fill that knowledge gap.

Having a trusted person who could inform them about services also allowed respondents to ask more sensitive questions, such as what impact their undocumented immigration status would have on their access to services. Some guiding figures were undocumented immigrants like themselves, but regardless of their immigration status, guiding figures played a crucial role in orienting immigrant women to different services.

Fortuitous Circumstances and Coethnic Ties

In addition to, or sometimes in lieu of, guiding figures, other means of gaining access to services were sometimes available to immigrant women, including proximity to nonprofit organizations and other coethnic ties through which they could be informed about services.

Hilda had migrated from Mexico to join her husband and adult daughter in a large city in the United States. For the first few months after she arrived, Hilda felt extremely isolated. She could not find work, and she had no connections to any organizations or institutions. One afternoon Hilda went for a walk to help ease her anxiety. Afraid of getting lost, she walked slowly and carefully, making sure to note the streets and signage around her. She happened to stop outside a community-based organization because its sign, which read CONSULTAS GRATIS (free consultations), grabbed her attention.

I came inside [the organization], and Dr. Marshall came out and asked me, "Are you looking for somebody who speaks Spanish?" I started crying. They said, "What's wrong? Sit down. Did something happen?" [I responded], "No, I just came from Mexico." "Don't worry," they said, "why don't you come to [the organization]? . . . We have lots of [resources]. If you want, tomorrow you can come, and we'll help you."

From that point on, Hilda visited the organization regularly, and throughout the years she developed a close rapport with its staff members, who had connected her to different kinds of informal-sector employment. Serendipitously accessing an organization, as Hilda did, is very rare, but it is noteworthy. Given the often unclear access to social services and hidden facades in suburban locations, as discussed in the previous chapter, it is clear that serendipitous encounters are more likely to happen in larger urban areas. Also noteworthy for Hilda was the protective function of being addressed in her native language; at this organization, she could communicate easily and felt more at ease explaining her situation. Other studies have shown that public-facing frontline staff can play a responsive role in welcoming recent immigrants into communities.[8] Other respondents described their encounters with fluent Spanish speakers as positive experiences that allowed them to become fully informed about the services they would receive.

Esperanza had only one acquaintance, Jose, when she first came to the United States, and he didn't prove to be very helpful in finding housing and employment. Thankfully, she was able to connect with Jose's friend Tony, who connected her to a job in a Mexican grocery store. She met her future husband at the grocery store and soon became pregnant with her first child. Her coethnic coworkers were the ones who instructed her to go to the WIC and Medi-Cal offices to sign up for services for herself and her child. Sofia's experience was similar. Asked how she found out about Medi-Cal and WIC after she became pregnant with her first child, Sofia said, "Well, I worked with four or five other [Latina] women. I would talk to them, and they would tell me about their experiences and where they had gone for [services]." For about one-third of respondents, coethnic coworkers, family members, or neighbors, noticing that they were pregnant or having trouble making ends meet, would inform them about organizations where they could receive aid. These neighbors and family members often went to these organizations themselves, so respondents were reassured that the aid they provided was feasible to receive and helpful.

Medical Need as a Condition to Seek Information

Having trustworthy and informed confidants was the best-case scenario for respondents in this study. Some respondents had uninformed or unsupportive networks that either were unable to inform them about available services or discouraged them from seeking much-needed services.

For example, Margarita's trajectory was very different from Judy's and Rosario's. She had not felt compelled to go to the United States so much as she was forced to by her parents. Her older sister was living in the United States without papers, and having recently left her abusive husband, she needed help taking care of her son. Her sister was uninformed about the services and supports available, so Margarita was similarly uninformed when she migrated north:

> When my sister was [in the United States], she worked as a single person for a long time taking care of children. . . . When she became pregnant, she continued to take care of children, and she never became informed about the type of aid she could receive for her son. She never asked. Nothing. She knew nothing . . . so when I came here, I didn't know that there was help for her son.

When Margarita became pregnant, she kept it hidden from her employer for as long as she could, and she also didn't go to the doctor during this time because her employer threatened to replace her if she missed a day of work. After asking her Spanish-speaking neighbors in her apartment complex, Margarita found out about a local free clinic she could go to and visited it five months into her pregnancy. While she was in the waiting room, another patient asked her in Spanish if she was on WIC. Margarita responded that she didn't know what that was, and the patient suggested that she ask her doctor about it. Margarita did, and soon she was able to sign up for the food assistance.

Five other respondents mentioned that they had found out about WIC, Medi-Cal, and other county-level health insurances (HealthPAC) for the first time when they went to a clinic for a pregnancy checkup and were informed there about these services. When I asked another respondent how she was able to sign up for Medi-Cal, she replied, "Medi-Cal? Really, [the clinic staff] did everything. They did everything. They told me they would give me insurance that would pay for everything, that I would qualify for it, and they did the entire process completely." In the absence of a guiding figure, these respondents became informed about available services through local clinics and hospitals.

One respondent's family, however, prevented her from accessing the local clinics and hospitals. Asunción migrated as a single mother in her forties to join her husband in Oakland. She moved into an unsupportive household and social network consisting of her in-laws and husband. Her in-laws took advantage of Asunción by expecting her to cook and provide free childcare, and her husband gave all his money to her in-laws, leaving none for her and her son. When I asked Asunción if she was aware of the availability of Medi-Cal or food stamps for her son when she first came here, she indicated that her husband never let her go to a clinic or ask for assistance in any form. He said that doing so would lower their chances of obtaining legal permanent resident status, and he didn't want any problems with *la migra* (immigration authorities).[9] Other respondents expressed similar concerns that, if they applied for food stamps or other public benefits for their children, they might ruin their chances of regularizing their immigration status in the future. Similar to Marta's concerns, as discussed in chapter 1, anxiety over proving themselves worthy of residency or citizenship in the future impacted their evaluation of whether they could safely prove themselves deserving of access to support for their basic needs in the present.

It wasn't until Asunción was facing a medical emergency that members of her prayer group convinced her to go to a free medical clinic, against her husband's advice. Finding that assistance was available there, Asunción returned to the clinic with her son and, through that clinic, applied for state health insurance and food assistance. In contrast to Judy and Rosario, Asunción had no guiding figures who led her through the different social services; instead, she found the help she needed through her connections to a prayer group whose members pushed her to seek services after her medical crisis arose. In other words, because of the influence of her unsupportive kin network, Asunción sought resources reactively rather than preemptively. Once her experience at the clinic made her feel safe, Asunción then had the confidence to participate in public benefit programs such as Medi-Cal and SNAP.

Institutional Openings to Primary Care

Gaining access to public programs not only gave immigrant women an institutional opening but motivated them to seek health care for themselves. Approximately 76 percent of undocumented respondents had found a venue for receiving primary care, and that percentage grew to 85 percent for documented women. Although these are not statistically representative statistics, they are indicative of immigrant women's access to primary care, which was different for the men in this study.

Women in Oakland were able to access primary care more easily than women in the suburbs, partly because of the higher number of FQHCs in Oakland. Women living in suburban areas had a much harder time finding a FQHC or free clinic. Rosario, for example, had the help of her neighbor Alma in gaining access to Medi-Cal and WIC, services that helped her take care of her children, but it took her a few more years to discover a primary care clinic for herself. She described the frustration in not finding a primary care clinic:

> Sometimes [I had], you know, a daily headache, and [I would ask myself], "Where do I make an appointment?" I would call the clinic, and [they would tell me], "This is only a women's clinic. Is this for prenatal care? If so, you can get an appointment. If not, then they won't accept you." So I asked myself, "Where? Where do I go?" And sometimes my husband would have something, and I would ask myself, "Where? Where do I go?"

Rosario kept asking acquaintances if they knew of places where she and her husband could be seen, and eventually a friend told her about a free clinic she went to and gave her a bulletin for it. Rosario called the clinic to schedule an appointment, but she was not able to get through. Her friend assured her that she would have to call several times to get through. The following week Rosario called for forty minutes straight until she was finally able to speak to a receptionist to get an appointment. She said that the effort was well worth it because she received good care there.

Rosario's narrative demonstrates that accessing primary care was a much less straightforward task for respondents than finding pregnancy-related services. Luckily for Rosario, she was able to find a primary care clinic that, though initially hard to reach, was available for needed care. Not all women were so lucky. Sofia, for example, did not know where to access primary care. When I asked her where she went when she got sick, she laughed and said, "I don't go anywhere! I self-diagnose. I say, 'Okay, I have vomiting; I have an infection.' If I go to the hospital, they'll probably give . . . amoxicillin, so I sometimes order my medicine [from Mexico]."

Other women felt left out of a system of care simply because of their immigration status. Asked where she went for medical services, Maria, a fifty-one-year-old mother of two, responded: "Sadly for me, there's nothing. . . . Obamacare is only for residents. It's so hard to find medical care [as an undocumented individual]. Before, there used to be more basic exams . . . at county clinics. Now they have reduced them because there's supposedly no funds. They're focused on getting [residents]. . . . They know they'll get money with them, you see?"

As other research indicates, Maria's difficulty in gaining access to health services signaled to her that she was an outsider who did not belong and was not deserving of care.[10] It was a feeling common among even those who did access services. As the previous chapter illustrated, some of the interactions in these settings were discriminatory and humiliating to immigrant women. Respondents preferred more specialized clinics for women or free health clinics run by community organizations over FQHCs. Although the men I interviewed accessed clinics and health care at a much lower rate than the women, they had the same preferences, perhaps because the care provided in community and specialty clinic settings was more culturally competent.

Moreover, the options available to uninsured and/or undocumented men and women were much narrower in suburban settings that had less experience of poverty. County-level programs for undocumented immigrants were available in Oakland, but many Alameda County municipalities cut programs that provided health services for undocumented immigrant adults after the foreclosure crisis in 2009 forced many budget cuts. Although a majority of the women in this study eventually accessed primary care, for all but one undocumented woman who was insured through her employer, health insurance was still out of reach. Health insurance was available only for their children. Even with the support of guiding figures, institutional mediators, and coethnic ties, political structures still prevented their access to high-quality, accessible care.

SOCIAL NETWORKS AND
RESOURCE-SEEKING PROCESSES

Scholars have long addressed the role of social networks in propelling people to migrate internationally.[11] For instance, some have examined Central American immigrants' estimation of their social networks as overly positive.[12] Other scholars have explored the positive and negative effects of ethnic neighborhoods in shaping access to local resources.[13] By underscoring the importance of informal, private ties in gaining both access to information about services and physical access to clinics, hospitals, and other social service institutions, I demonstrate here the power of bonding ties in resource-finding behavior. "Bonding ties" refers to the sharing of similar traits with another person—the point of bonding between people.[14] Bonding ties contrast with "bridging ties," which are heterogenous ties that have been conceptualized as "bridging" people to new networks or resources. Bonding ties are typically characterized as drivers of social inclusion, but they are typically *not* conceptualized as ties that connect to new resources. This study, in highlighting the importance of bonding ties for connecting individuals to resources suggested by people who are trusted, knowledgeable, and experienced sources of information, adds nuance to past research that underscored the importance of bridging ties for low-income individuals.[15]

Research on NPOs highlights their role in expanding individuals' social capital and acting as a catalyst for collective mobilization.[16] Less attention has been paid, however, to the *initial* social capital that facilitates access to these institutions. Understanding how individuals originally access NPOs can help these organizations establish better outreach to low-income and immigrant populations. Moreover, understanding how individuals decide to claim public benefits would complement research that emphasizes the political nature of this claiming process. Joe Soss frames claiming welfare benefits as a form of "survival politics" that can complement more collective, confrontational politics to effect broader change.[17] A similar narrative of resource-seeking as political action appears in the immigration literature. For example, Kathleen Coll describes the "good information" (*buena información*) provided through the NPO Mujeres, Unidas, y Activas (MUA) as one of the first steps taken toward the politicization of the undocumented women who "remade citizenship" in San Francisco in the mid-1990s.[18] Armed with information on navigating and advocating for their children in state institutions, women can become more empowered and savvier as they pursue other resources and pass along their knowledge to others. Although some scholarship has downplayed the potential of increased political participation through informal network support among individuals experiencing poverty, this scholarship is not explicitly focused on immigrant populations, among whom learning the bureaucratic ropes of an institution can serve as a bridge to civic engagement more generally.[19]

UNDERSTANDING CONDITIONAL SAFETY

In the absence of federal immigration reform, "conditional safety" can be found in the spaces and processes that enable and provide access to services for undocumented immigrants, who face the risk of being deported and separated from their children, from their spouses, and from a country they have worked hard to establish themselves in. In this study, how respondents perceived their risk of deportation varied widely, but they all acknowledged it as a real possibility they had to face. Finding spaces where their immigration status would not be used against them (at least not immediately) allowed undocumented women to take the risk of disclosing their status to one person or another. Once they found conditionally safe spaces, they were able to form bonds with other women, find other resources, and breathe a bit easier knowing that their children did not have to go hungry or forgo medical care.

The concept of "conditional safety" that I have developed in this book is sorely needed in immigration literature, which tends to emphasize "legal violence" and to pay less attention to the strategies used to mitigate it. The concept of conditional safety could also be expanded and applied to scholarship that focuses on other marginalized populations, such as unhoused populations or individuals with a criminal record who are negatively impacted by laws that limit where they can live or the public benefits they can receive.[20] Like undocumented immigrants, these are marginalized populations who are often stigmatized as undeserving of care or access to services and may also rely on institutions or informal strategies to uplift themselves.

As we have seen in this chapter, currently or formerly undocumented women are most often in contact with public institutions related to the health and education of their children.[21] These women's networks guide them through the different services available to them, but this did not happen for the undocumented men I interviewed. Men do guide other men toward employment and inform them of English classes, but when they enter the medical system, undocumented men are most likely to do so through an employer or when they are prompted to seek help in a medical emergency. Most of the immigrant men I interviewed, however, never sought out medical care at all. Even if they had access to insurance through an employer, they reported having never gone to a clinic in all the years they had lived in the United States. In discussing immigrant men's experiences accessing social services—or not—in the following chapter, I show how structural conditions and a culture of masculinity intersect to reinforce the limited conditions under which they have access to services and care.

CHAPTER 4

"I Don't Have Anything. No Doctor . . . No Nothing": Labor and Crises as Conditions for Care

On a warm Tuesday evening in the fall, I walked into a day labor center in Oakland to introduce the interview project to a group of about twenty men and five women. This day labor center was unlike the others I had visited. It also served as a community health clinic that offered food assistance, free therapy sessions by licensed mental health clinicians, and social service referrals to city, county, and state programs. Five minutes before the meeting started, the room was already full of older adults who had clearly finished a day of work: their T-shirts and jeans were stained with paint, and the expressions on some faces were weary.

But not Manuel. Manuel stood out from the other workers because of his white hair, taller figure, lean frame, and kind eyes that always seemed to be smiling. When I explained the project to the people in the room, Manuel sat up in rapt attention while others slumped in their seats from fatigue. He was the first person to approach me after the meeting to express interest in an interview, and we quickly settled on a time the following week. The day before our meeting, Manuel called to apologize and ask if we could reschedule for later in the week. His employer had just offered him work, and he needed to take it.

We met one morning at the center and settled into a small room sometimes used for mental health counseling. There was just enough space for myself, the research assistant accompanying me that day, and Manuel, who sat facing me across a small circular table. The staff at the day labor center had made the effort to make this small room look as cheery as possible; it was painted bright orange, with decorative Día de Los Muertos skeletons on the walls and a vase with a plastic rose sitting atop the small table. The room clearly aimed to welcome Latinx immigrants by communicating some semblance of "home."

Manuel wore a long-sleeved white shirt and jeans and looked older than his fifty-six years. His skin was weathered, and his hands had dried white paint on them, the residue of his previous two days of work. He carried a stack of loose-leaf notebook papers that visibly shook in his hand. I later learned that the papers contained his testimony statement—written in elegant cursive handwriting—to being the victim of a domestic crime. A group of men had severely beaten him one night, and now he was applying for a U-visa.

To lighten the mood we talked a bit about the weather, and he told me about the job he had just secured for a few days. He expressed his relief at having multiday work because stable employment was hard to come by. Indeed, Manuel was living in a state of financial precarity. The structural vulnerability of his situation, over which he had little control, had left him frustrated and desperate as he engaged in a complicated search for resources and aid.

Manuel had come to the United States in the early 1990s seeking work to pay his children's tuition expenses, which were unaffordable for him on his *campesino* (fieldworker) wages. Manuel had expected the trip to be temporary, but he had not returned to Mexico even once. Manuel had not seen his family in over twenty years. Making things more difficult was that he had not formed a new family in the United States. When I asked if he had any family when he first came here, he said, "No, even to this day. No wife, no sons. I only came with my friends." His friends were other men he knew from his hometown. They all came to the United States to seek whatever employment they could find.

Once they had settled in Oakland, Manuel and his acquaintances decided to meet at street corners to wait for work; they also kept each other informed of important resources and services they could access, like housing opportunities and food assistance. During those years, work was abundant, but so were laborers. Everybody had to act quickly to get a job amid such tight competition. For the past two decades, Manuel had worked as a day laborer, moving from one corner to another in Oakland for work, and from one crowded apartment complex to the next for housing.

Several months after arriving in the United States, Manuel found out about a community-based organization that offered free meals and information about where to find employment at fair wages. He also took English and computer classes at the center and proudly talked about receiving a diploma for completing computer classes. That accomplishment reminded him of his painstaking efforts to help his children receive high school diplomas.

Despite having access to the worker center and its services, Manuel had still hung on by a thin financial thread. The thread had become even thinner when he was injured at work several years ago. While working on a last-minute side job, he fell through a roof and gravely injured his leg. His employer—an acquaintance of his—had no insurance and simply handed him some cash as he was rushed off to the hospital. In the end, the county's emergency medical insurance covered Manuel's medical expenses, and through connections with a labor lawyer, he received money from the city in which he worked and resided to compensate for his broken leg. But the aftereffects of the injury endured, and the small sum of money Manuel received from the city had not stabilized his financial situation. After a second workplace injury, Manuel had been unable to afford chiropractic sessions to restore his mobility.

To make matters worse, Manuel had chronic tooth pain, and despite his best efforts, he had been unsuccessful in finding affordable dental care. Manuel had no choice but to work through the pain; it was the only way to ensure his subsistence. After expressing his concerns about rising rent, he explained, "Today I don't have work, I don't earn [money]. It's been fifteen days since I've worked, and I've been spending money [on food]. Right now, I only have $150 for rent, but my reassurance is that I still have more money coming from two and a half days of work, so that helps me sleep at night." He then detailed his careful calculation of his daily, weekly, and monthly living expenses.

By excluding undocumented populations from safe, stable work, the formal U.S. labor market forces them into informal work that damages their health, creating a vicious cycle: undocumented men must work to sustain themselves, but once they are injured, their physical health is weakened, their ability to work is impaired, and they are coerced into a state of simply trying to survive. With limited networks, and being undocumented, Manuel had been funneled into this extremely precarious informal labor market featuring physically laborious and injury-prone work. His two injuries and aging body were making it more difficult to continue this work and thus to sustain himself. Not all workers I interviewed had experienced hardship as severe as Manuel's. Nevertheless, his situation served as a cautionary tale of what happens in an economic regime that prioritizes labor and devalues health.

Both men and women who are undocumented have limited access to social services and health care, but as I show in this chapter, their challenges in accessing and receiving services differ. As detailed in the preceding chapter, one of undocumented women's most significant barriers to accessing services was their fear that their immigration status would not only make them ineligible for programs but later be used against them or their family members as they sought to regularize their immigration status. Pregnant women and women who were mothers, however, met the policy conditions necessary to be eligible for programs like WIC and Medi-Cal. Women's coethnic networks provided a second condition for accessing services. Having overcome the initial hurdle of accessing care, women had a relatively broader institutional entrée into social services and health care based on their gendered role as a mother. Although they were initially afraid and hesitant to sign up for services, the state gave mothers a clear structural opening into services—an opening culturally reinforced by the social networks that helped them to seek services and to feel less shame in doing so.

By contrast, men faced greater structural and cultural limitations when they sought out resources and services. On a macro-structural level, undocumented men, unlike women, had no access to public programs like WIC or Medi-Cal and therefore lacked a clear opening to services. The only condition they could meet to gain access to public services was having a medical crisis. Reinforcing this highly conditional access was a self-narrative of masculinity and an immigrant work ethic, both of which served these men to some degree as ways to cope with not having access to a highly conditional safety net. The men I interviewed claimed not to need care (which they could not access). They said that they never got sick or needed to go to a doctor and that they used health services only in emergency medical situations.

For some men, however, their search for employment unexpectedly led them to seek primary or preventative care. As men informed each other about employment opportunities, they found out about worker centers. Apart from providing access to fair-wage employment, these centers offered information and connections to health-related services, including food assistance, clinics, and county health programs, thus mitigating some of the barriers to health care and services for the men who walked through their doors. Thus, the policy conditions that enabled undocumented men to access services were very limited (namely, having coverage through an employer or facing a medical crisis), and the practical condition that allowed some to eventually access services was very narrow (being connected to services through worker centers). Under these narrow conditions, men had much more limited access than women to the safety net, both in policy and in practice.

CONTEXTUALIZING MEN'S POORER HEALTH AND LOWER HEALTH CARE USAGE

Public health and social network scholars have long documented gender differences in health and health care access. One possible cause of these differences is the shape and form of men's and women's networks. In general terms, cisgender heterosexual men benefit more from marriage than cisgender heterosexual women because their wives have a positive influence on their health behaviors.[1] Men are also less likely to seek health resources than women, even when they need it most.[2] Some of the differences in health care usage have been attributed in this literature to a culture of masculinity that encourages men to ignore pain or to underestimate the severity of negative symptoms or diagnoses. This socialization often leads them to seek care less often than women, or to seek it too late for effective treatment.[3] This literature does little to complicate notions of masculinity, as it assumes that men adhere to a hegemonic masculinity and does not discuss male populations that may contest it.[4]

Studies that have made comparisons within male populations have found that in the United States men of lower socioeconomic status (SES) have poorer health outcomes than higher-SES men; they have also found that Latino and Black men are less likely to seek health resources than White men and Latina or Black women.[5] This disparity grows when it comes to accessing mental health care services.[6] Because most of this literature is quantitative and survey-based, it provides less insight into the impact of structural barriers to health care on men's access to and usage of health care services. These structural barriers, however, are especially pertinent to low-income and undocumented populations.

The Role of Immigration Status in Men's Health

Turning to the impact of immigration status on health, we find consensus on the significant barriers that undocumented populations face in accessing health care. To begin with, a majority of the undocumented population in California (70 percent) is estimated to have income under 200 percent of the federal poverty line, and of those earning under that income, an estimated 41 percent are uninsured.[7] These estimates coincide with estimates from national-level data that 42 percent of the undocumented population is uninsured.[8] These percentages and numbers are expected to only grow with an aging immigrant population.[9] And in the United States, uninsured populations have much less access to health care overall.[10] This is a problem that impacts not only immigrants but the 8 percent of U.S. citizens who were uninsured as of 2020.[11] Additionally, undocumented migrants disproportionately work in the informal labor force, where they are subject to dismal work and health conditions. Historically, immigrant laborers have experienced labor exploitation, employer intimidation, and dangerous working conditions in physically arduous jobs. Earning low and often irregular wages, immigrants are also forced by their limited economic resources into subpar and potentially dangerous housing conditions. In these circumstances, many develop chronic health problems and suffer work injuries.

In *Fresh Fruit: Broken Bodies*, the anthropologist Seth Holmes describes the living conditions of undocumented Latinx workers in the agriculture industry in Washington State. In one location Holmes visited, nineteen people lived in a three-bedroom apartment; for at least a month and sometimes longer, they worked twelve to eighteen hours a day, six to seven days a week.[12] Surveys of agricultural workers indicate that they suffer from a slew of chronic health conditions and diseases caused by their backbreaking manual labor in the fields. They develop chemical- or pesticide-related illnesses, numerous skin conditions, respiratory conditions, and musculoskeletal disorders as they endure daily chronic pain and headaches.[13] However, employers dismiss workers' concerns about pain or medical conditions and respond dismissively with the racist claim that Indigenous bodies are equipped to endure more pain.[14] According to a Center for Urban Economic Development report on day laborers, "One in five day laborers has suffered a work-related injury, and more than half of those who were injured in the past year did not receive medical care."[15]

The devaluation of immigrants' health has deep historical roots. From the time that immigrant populations started to become a part of the U.S. workforce, the state has largely been concerned for immigrants' health only insofar as it contributes to their productivity and labor. With the passage of the Immigration Act in 1891, any person stepping on U.S. soil had to undergo a health inspection to ensure that they did not carry a "loathsome or a dangerous contagious disease."[16] Although the mandate made sense for protecting public health, in 1903 the true purpose of the medical inspections was revealed.

Even immigrants with no condition that would pose a public health threat to others were turned back by the Public Health Service if they had diseases or conditions that would limit them from working to their full potential. They were labeled as "likely to become a public charge" and swiftly denied admission at the border. Immigrants had to prove their labor potential to the United States in order to enter the country; no "sick," "ill," or even pregnant immigrants were allowed.[17] This project to prevent the influx of immigrants seen as "unfit" was tied in part to the eugenics movement, which framed itself as "racial hygiene" and heavily influenced public policies, from immigration to health. California had some of the most sweeping eugenics laws in the nation and was the third state to adopt forced sterilization in 1909,[18] some of which were carried out on Latinx immigrants.[19]

During the typhus outbreak in Los Angeles in 1917, Mexican agricultural workers and other Mexicans who wanted to cross the U.S. border had to strip for nude inspections and bathe in gasoline to get rid of lice that could spread the typhus. Forced inspection and fumigation were paired with a psychological examination as well as questions about visa and citizenship status, and the arms of workers were even tattooed with the word ADMITTED as a mark of cleanliness. Many of the public officials who designed this response to typhus had been active participants in state eugenics and public health initiatives.[20] Because unsanitary conditions were prominent in the agricultural work camps where many Mexicans worked, the disease was attributed to Mexicans for being "dirty" instead of to employers for exploiting workers and providing poor housing conditions that compromised their health. These fumigation practices continued well in the 1950s for Mexican braceros. These contract workers were sprayed with dangerous chemicals like DDT and other insecticides to "delouse" them.[21] Immigrant health was not only devalued but pathologized.

In describing the relationship between immigrant men's labor and their health, this book does not mean to understate the heavy toll that work can take on women. Undocumented immigrant women engaged in informal employment as caretakers and cleaners are subject to low wages, verbal and sexual abuse, and toxic chemicals that can harm their health. A 2007 collaborative report by Oakland nonprofit organizations found that 95 percent of household workers were uninsured, and that 64 percent did not seek medical care for injuries or illnesses.[22] Both men and women face exploitative labor conditions that limit their access to health care. Moreover, their immigration status, especially in combination with racial discrimination, can lead to health disparities for immigrants over time.[23] In examining why they did not receive medical care, the study revealed that most undocumented workers cannot afford health care and employers often do not provide health insurance for these workers. Workers themselves, already living on a minimal budget, must assume responsibility for any medical expenses they incur.

At the same time, the physically heavy toll of their work is often a source of pride for undocumented workers, particularly for men. It comes as no surprise that many immigrant men embrace their identities as strong, invincible workers with no need for medical treatment given that the limited positive discourse on immigrants focuses on their roles as laborers, men are largely excluded from public health care, and a culture of masculinity tells them that voicing pain is a sign of weakness. This message can be reinforced by employers' false allegations that differently racialized bodies naturally endure varying levels of pain.[24] Undocumented workers' commitment to a strong, self-disciplinary ethic and investment in their identity as laborers may underlie their reluctance to report unhealthy working conditions or unfair wages in the workplace, despite the legal right of undocumented workers to workplace protections, including a right to work breaks and to paid time for their reported hours, worker's compensation, protection from discrimination, and the right to union membership, among others.[25] Real structural barriers insidiously shape and reinforce a culture of masculinity. As a result of long-standing structural violence, vulnerable populations internalize an external oppression. Undocumented men are relegated to informal, exploitative labor markets that worsen their health while simultaneously excluding them from access to comprehensive medical care. Even those who are aware of the medical options hypothetically available to them do not seek care because the financial cost of that care remains too high. The men in this study rarely used health services and usually did so only in the event of a severe medical crisis or work injury.

UNDOCUMENTED MEN'S HIGHLY CONDITIONAL ACCESS TO CARE

In the previous chapter, I detailed how, despite their undocumented immigration status, women in this study, seeking care for their children, were generally able to access some health services through public programs like Medi-Cal and WIC as well as other services like food assistance and educational classes. Their access to health care for themselves was neither perfect nor easy, but through the support of guiding figures, coethnic ties, and institutional referrals,

77 percent of these undocumented women reported being connected to and using primary care.

The picture for undocumented men in the study looked quite different, with only 35 percent reporting access to a source of primary care. Because they were unable to access broad public programs like WIC (unless they were the sole custodial parent or guardian of a young child) and were not eligible for Medi-Cal coverage for non-emergency or non-pregnancy-related health care, they had no clear institutional opening into services. Because most undocumented men work in the informal labor market, they also had no access to health insurance. I argue that the lower rate of primary care knowledge and usage among men is due in part to access barriers. These barriers make it difficult to find out about primary care; combined with extremely constrained health care options, this lack of knowledge makes undocumented populations even more reluctant to try to access care at all.

Encountering Conditional Care

Jorge's experience offers a good place to begin explaining the barriers to health care faced by men with liminal immigration status. A day laborer in his early fifties and father of two adult children, Jorge was born in El Salvador and had migrated to Oakland about eighteen years earlier. Like Manuel, Jorge was a prospective interviewee I met at the day labor center in Oakland. Although he also expressed enthusiasm for an interview, he had a fatigued, almost despondent demeanor. He was tired of his physically arduous job, and when I met with him, he apologized for his appearance—paint fumes irritated his reddened eyes, and white paint splattered his worn blue jeans.

Jorge had been one of the eldest of twelve siblings. His father worked in *el campo* (as a fieldworker) harvesting crops, while his mother was a homemaker. Jorge was only able to attend elementary school through third grade before he started working odd jobs to help his family make ends meet. Later he sold and bought livestock, and in his early twenties he got married and had two daughters. When his daughters were six and nine years old, Jorge took advantage of an opportunity that arose to go to California and earn money so that he could provide more money for his family. After six years of painting for a company that his nephew had connected him to in San Francisco, Jorge left to join his niece washing cars in a rural central California town. One year later, he moved to Oakland, joining two other nephews in the restaurant industry.

Jorge worked Thursday through Monday at a restaurant and went to the day labor center to pick up painting and construction work on the other days. He did not enjoy the physically grueling nature of his work, but painting and construction were the skills he had to use to subsist in Oakland and to chip in for his family's expenses in El Salvador. His situation made it difficult for Jorge to access information on the limited health care options available to him. When I asked him where he went if he became ill, he said that he had seen a doctor only twice in the past sixteen years. Both times were serendipitous and happened when he passed by pharmacies that advertised free medical consultations in his Oakland neighborhood. He wanted insurance, but he didn't know what options were available to him as someone with temporary protected status (TPS).

In addition to their lack of information on the limited health care to which their immigration status gave them access, the restrictedness of the options they did have deterred these men from even trying to seek care at all. In other words, these conditions had the chilling effect of encouraging them to preemptively make no attempt to seek health care, out of the (often correct) suspicion that they would not be eligible for low-cost care. Because undocumented men feared that they could not afford the cost of medical care, they would wait until an emergency arose before seeking treatment at a public hospital.

Manuel, for example, did not know where to go for affordable care, and the thought of paying full cost for medical services stressed him out and made him anxious. When I asked Manuel if he had health insurance, he said, "No, no, no, no. No, no. (*stammering*) I don't have anything. No doctor . . . no nothing." But then Manuel claimed, "I mean, I've never gotten sick, thank God. The only time [I did], I went directly to a [public hospital], and the other time, that I had tooth pain—it's horrible to sit with that pain." In claiming never to have been sick—except for those two emergency situations—Manuel seemed to be trying to categorically rule out the possibility that he would ever need expensive medical services.

In another interview, Eddie, a fifty-year-old day laborer living in Oakland and father of an adult child, said that he thought he had health insurance, but he wasn't sure. When I asked him for more information, he said that he had gone to the public hospital for a medical emergency and that a "counsel" person there had helped him register for a Medi-Cal card for low-income people. With this card, he didn't have to pay any medical bills. He had received the card several years earlier, however, and had made no attempt to renew his registration and get a replacement card. When I asked Eddie if he knew about the doctors connected to the worker center he was a part of, he responded that he had a checkup when he joined the center five years earlier but had not had a checkup since then. I probed for reasons why, but the closest I got to an answer from Eddie was that he simply didn't prioritize making health care appointments because he was most concerned about having work. For men working as day laborers or landscapers, their highly irregular employment in the informal labor market makes it difficult for them to spend time waiting in clinics or seeking out information on how to access services and resources, including medical care.

Coping with Conditional Care

Faced with limited health care access, the men in the study used different strategies to cope with insufficient care. Downplaying their need for medical care was one strategy; emphasizing their agency and ability to maintain their health was another. When I asked Ronaldo, a fifty-seven-year-old landscaper and father of one, where he went if he got sick, he responded, "I go nowhere. . . . I try to avoid a doctor because it's really expensive." Then he animatedly explained that cutting down on red meat in his diet kept him healthy and his physical labor kept him strong. Soon after discussing his healthy habits, however, he admitted, "The only thing that bothers me is that I had an accident in Mexico, and I hurt my back. . . . I saw a chiropractor here [in the United States] . . . but it was too expensive; I had to end the treatment because I couldn't pay it. . . . But other than that, I'm healthy."

Undocumented, Ronaldo worked odd jobs to make ends meet. He had no insurance from his employer, and no access to countywide health services. Despite the structural barriers to health care he faced, Ronaldo emphasized his agency—how he took care of his own health was the general theme throughout the interview. He wanted to maintain a positive attitude, believed in the meritocratic myth of the United States, and did not want his immigration status to drag him down. Toward the end of the interview, he said, "With papers or without papers, you can prosper in this country." Ronaldo knew he had value in the United States, and he did not critique the broader structures that impeded his access to proper health care.

Jesús, echoing Ronaldo's emphasis on personal agency, was determined not to let his undocumented status undermine his experiences in the United States. He had risked using a fake Social Security number to secure employment at different places that all offered him health insurance. But again, he did not seek preventative medical care even though he had access to primary health care. He claimed to have never gotten sick or gone to a doctor in his six years in the country. At the time of our interview, he was visibly sick, chronically coughing and blowing his nose. When I asked him if he would prefer to schedule the interview for another time, he insisted on continuing, even though he was scheduled to work a shift at the restaurant where he was employed afterward.[26]

Pablo exemplified the strategy of not seeking medical care until injured. A day laborer and father of three who had resided in Concord for fourteen years, Pablo was originally from a large city in Mexico. Like many other men in this study, he went north to work in order to supplement his family's income. He had children to support, and he deeply cared about their well-being. Pablo went back and forth between Mexico and Concord three times in four years because he found it painful to be away from his children for too long.

On his third trip north, he brought his children with him. Pablo's gentle voice and calm demeanor belied the trauma he endured crossing the desert with them twelve years earlier. Now his children were grown and doing well, and he lived with his oldest son and daughter-in-law in their apartment. He worked for a contractor most days and went to a day labor center on rainy days to find work. Pablo seemed fit and spry for his forty-six years, but that didn't preclude his need for medical services. When I asked Pablo where he went if he had a medical problem, he answered:

> Well, before, I had basic [health] care. . . . But in 2009, they took away the basic care service for immigrants, with the crisis and the [budget] cuts. The state realized that there were a lot of immigrants with basic [health] care, and they took it away. They only left us with emergency health care. . . . The good thing is that I don't get sick, so I haven't had to see a doctor up until now.[27]

When I followed up and asked whether he would go to a doctor when he became sick or if he had a problem with his health, he replied, "I don't get sick. I've only gone—for example, one time I hurt myself at work, and I went to Martinez [the public hospital]. Because I had emergency health care, they attended me there."

In all of these examples, undocumented men claimed that they never got sick and did not need medical care. They sought help, despite the high costs potentially involved, only in medical emergencies, such as when they were injured. Their first response to questions about health care was to downplay their need for medical services to which, in any event, they had no easy access. That lack of access to primary care had serious negative implications for them.

Primary Health Care: The Dangers of Conditionality

Lack of access to preventative care has all kinds of dangerous consequences, from not seeking medical care for a problem that becomes an emergency to suffering the complications of having manageable but long-untreated chronic conditions like high cholesterol and diabetes. Ramón, whom I spoke about in chapter 1, decided to forgo medical care after robbers assaulted him at a Home Depot. In another example, Rodrigo could not have surgery for a hernia for fifteen years because it was not considered an emergency that would be covered by insurance for low-income patients. Not until a worker center staff member enrolled him in a countywide health services program did Rodrigo finally obtain the surgery.

I witnessed how important it was to have access to clinic-based preventative care through my participant observation as a volunteer in a local clinic for uninsured patients. When patients came in with symptoms that, on their own, would not be considered urgent—like severe, persistent headaches or faint numbness developing in the hands—the clinic doctors were able to connect these symptoms to potentially harmful conditions, like the onset of a facial stroke or severe diabetes that needed to be managed. Doctors referred a couple of patients to an emergency department at a nearby hospital for immediate treatment. If doctors or nurses detected high diabetes or cholesterol levels, they offered medicine to lower blood sugar or cholesterol and follow-up with free one-on-one consultations on diabetes education and management.

When I asked male patients how they found out about the clinic, many said that their family members or friends had told them about it. The men I interviewed for this study, however, did not mention this medical clinic, suggesting that information on free local clinics was not widely shared, especially among men.

FINDING CRASH PADS: EMPLOYMENT
AS AN INDIRECT VEHICLE TO CARE

So far this chapter has delineated the barriers and challenges that immigrant men face in accessing health care and the resulting dangers to their health and sometimes even their survival. Given the obstacles these men are up against, how do they eventually access care?

Surprisingly enough, employment had provided many men in the study with a link to care. Their social networks had helped connect them to employment in the first place. In other words, men openly shared information on work, and some men thus found out about worker centers, where they were connected to day labor opportunities at fair wages. The worker centers would also inform them about health services or help them sign up for different services. While pregnancy gave women a more direct path to referrals to clinics and other resources, men had a much more convoluted, but at times successful, path to primary care.

"One Day I Came into the United States, and the Next Day I Was Working": Coethnic Information Sharing on Employment

One of the main reasons men immigrated was to seek higher-paying work opportunities that would grant them and their families a better life than they could afford in their country of origin. Thus, work was of utmost importance to them upon arriving in the United States. Fortunately, information on finding work was relatively easy to come by. Some men secured stable employment with the employers of their friends and family members. Other men forged alliances with people in similar situations and traded information on how to get access to work in the informal labor market. While the stability and nature of work differed slightly for the men in this study, the common thread among their experiences was the role of coethnic, often gendered, networks in helping them secure employment.

Jesús, whom I mentioned earlier in the chapter and described in chapter 1, was born in the large city of Guadalajara, where he grew up as the eldest of six sons. After finishing secondary school, Jesús helped support his family, along with his father. In his early twenties Jesús married and he and his wife had their only child. At the insistence of his wife's older brother, who had migrated to the United States, Jesús and his wife and child joined him there in 2005.

Through his brother-in-law, Jesús was immediately able to get a job. "My [wife's] brother worked in a [construction] company," Jesús said, "and right away, when he found out we were coming, he talked to his supervisor and [said], 'Look, my brother-in-law is coming.' 'Yes, bring him in,' [his supervisor said]. . . . One day we came [to the United States], and the next day I was working." Ten other men told similar stories of a male family member connecting them to a job right away in construction, the restaurant industry, or landscaping. Anyone who didn't have the skill set for a particular job learned on the job. For example, when I asked Oscar how he obtained work upon coming to the United States, he responded, "[My friends] helped me. They worked as landscapers. I didn't have any experience in it, but they taught me how to landscape." Friends as well as family members helped orient and support incoming immigrants by sharing living spaces and crucial information.

Gerardo initially resided in California's Central Valley. When I asked him how he started to search for jobs, he said, "There are friends who tell you, 'Go to this place,' and there's work." He initially had trouble finding work in factories because of his limited English skills, but soon he was able to locate a temporary agency that dispatched him to different jobs.

Because he had legal permanent residency, Gerardo was eligible to work for the agency. Men relegated to the informal labor market said that they would hear about certain street corners where work was handed out and they would head there together. For example, Jorge started looking for work on street corners in Berkeley even though he lived in Oakland. When I asked him why, he said, "Through my friends, they told me it was good. Really good, because there, if we didn't get work, organizations would come by and give us lunch." Manuel also found out about a day labor organization through his friends. "I would wait on street corners, and [organization staff] would let us know that an organization existed there . . . and they had food." Manuel and his friends would walk from the street corner to the day labor center, where, besides employment opportunities, they would find out about services and resources available to them.

Workplace Interventions as Conditions to Access Care

About one-quarter of the men in the study—even those who had lived and worked in the United States for many years—were connected to health services for the first time when they joined a worker center. Because Oakland is located in Alameda County, undocumented day laborers at the worker center in Oakland could get access to the HealthPAC program, which gave them access to basic health services and care. At the Concord location, however, the free county health service program was less robust. The Contra Costa Cares program provided free health services at four medical sites for up to three thousand low-income residents on a first-come, first-served basis. But because the county cut funding for primary care services for undocumented adults in 2009, most of the men in the study were under the impression that no primary care options were available to them in the county. One outlet for needed care that they typically were informed about was a federally qualified health center, which required membership to receive services. Members could also be referred to the Contra Costa Cares program.

Carlos's experience in learning about low-cost health-care clinics was typical. He was a day laborer who had immigrated to Concord from El Salvador a month before the interview. Asked if he had found out about any food or medical services, Carlos said that just the day before the staff members talked about it at the worker center he went to. "The staff told us we had centers where we could go for a [low-cost] medical consultation. For me, that's good. It's a good help because getting sick is really expensive. The best thing is not to get sick, but one isn't in charge of that, illnesses come of their own accord." Carlos didn't recall the name of the clinic that was recommended to him, but if he wanted or needed medical attention, he knew he could reach out to center staff or other center members for advice on where to go for care. Although men in the study did not always seek care when they needed it, at least knowing where they could go for services made it more likely that they would frequent a health care clinic, nonprofit organization, or public hospital if the need for care continued or worsened.

Worker Centers as Resource Hubs   Although workers were initially attracted to worker centers for the food and work opportunities provided there, they soon learned about other services they could access through either the center or other organizations. They found out about food pantries, English classes, computer classes, medical clinics, and health service programs like HealthPAC in Alameda County.

Workers who knew about the center would then refer their friends to it and share information about what was available. Although not everyone liked the center, some decided to stay. In a rare case, Rodrigo brought a friend into the center to seek not merely a work opportunity but also treatment for his diabetes at an on-site clinic. "I wanted to show him the place," Rodrigo said. "Even though they had told him that he could look for work here and they told him that there's a clinic to help treat his diabetes, I brought him here, so I can directly show him the place."

Another day laborer, Vicente, reported that his hometown acquaintances oriented him to different resources and services available in the town. "When

I first came [to the United States], the first thing my friends told me is where the adult school was to learn English, where the work center was, where stores were [located]," he said. Vicente's friends also assured him "that the police wasn't immigration, so there was no need to hide from the police."[28] Through the day labor center, he then found out about a FQHC and a food pantry. He joined the FQHC and seeks food assistance at the food pantry as needed.

The experiences of Vicente and Rodrigo's friend illustrate not only the operation of organizations as referral hubs and sources of critical resources but also the role of coethnic networks in securing those resources. Thus, many men in this study fortuitously turned up opportunities to learn about health care and other resources when they sought work. In the absence of worker centers, however, and for anything other than a medical emergency, referrals to health care services were much harder for them to come by.

STEPPING BACK: THE ROLE OF PLACE AND LARGER CULTURAL NARRATIVES

This chapter has made clear that undocumented men are up against tremendous obstacles to seeking and accessing health care. Unlike the women I spoke to, they had no clear institutional opening into public programs, like WIC and non-emergency Medi-Cal, through parental status or pregnancy, and they often worked in physically arduous jobs at irregular hours, for irregular wages, and with no employer insurance. Compounding their situation was a lack of time or resources to access information about the already limited health care to which they did have access.

The obstacles are high for women as well, but they often have the critical backing of other women as they navigate the information barriers. Men's coethnic networks support them and share information on resources, but the types of resources they share are primarily employment-related. Women are also given referrals to employment, but the difference between women and most men is that women refer each other to *both* employment opportunities and health care sites. Most men access information on medical care only after they have a medical emergency or when a worker center provides them with information on clinics, health service or insurance programs, and on-site medical care (if available). Fortunately, some men in the study joined worker centers that offered such information.

Yet worker centers can apply only a small bandage to the structural violence reproduced by the larger system. As Manuel's story shows at the beginning of this chapter, even with access to a worker center, an undocumented man suffering from chronic conditions, such as back and tooth pain, has no access to low-cost specialized services through which he can be treated, like chiropractic or dental services. Despite belonging to a worker center, Manuel was faced with worsening health and financial instability. Moreover, his worker center was exceptional; most worker centers do not host on-site health care clinics or provide wraparound services like referrals, food assistance, and language classes. Furthermore, as noted in chapter 2, there are considerable differences in the kinds of resources available to undocumented men and women depending on the city, county, and state in which they live.

For broader systemic change to occur, the narrative on immigrants' health must be humanized. Immigrants' health should matter not only because healthy immigrants bring labor and economic benefits to the country but also because, like anyone else, immigrants have a right to health. This right to health care must include both emergency and preventative care, and it cannot be contingent on narrow qualifiers on who deserves access to health services. As the next chapter demonstrates, today undocumented immigrants are challenging the public discourse that stigmatizes Latinx immigrants as unwanted (and undeserving) individuals subject to deportation. They recognize their value not only as laborers but as a population deserving of dignity, regardless of their immigration status. They should not have to prove their economic, educational, or financial worth to exercise their right to health, and this right to health should not be dependent on immigration status.

CHAPTER 5

"We Give the Best to the Country, but the Country Is Not Ready to Give the Best to Us": Engaging the Logic of Conditional Care

Magdalena was at her wits' end. The years of work she put into earning an education degree in Mexico turned out to be of no use in the United States. She wanted to pursue her passion for teaching while earning an income to help support her family, but because she was undocumented, she couldn't do that. Instead, she invested in her children and their schooling by enrolling them in supplementary educational programs, and she also took on some English classes herself. Slowly but surely, she became more involved in community-based organizations and found out about more resources and opportunities for herself and her family. When she learned that a nonprofit was offering to subsidize courses at a community college for low-income adults, Magdalena saw a chance to earn the credentials she needed to teach in the United States.

At the information session about the program held at the nonprofit, Magdalena learned that she needed to have a Social Security number to be eligible for the subsidized courses. She remembered exclaiming, "It's not fair! . . . I have my rights too, and I don't always want to be low-income." Furious, she told her friends about her situation, and the friends advised her that not having a Social Security number might not be an issue if she enrolled in person at the college. "I went with my stroller and my children, and they never asked me for my Social [Security]. I don't know if they overlooked it, if they forgot, but they gave me my student number." Magdalena, like other respondents, spoke out about the injustice of a system that restricted the upward mobility of people simply because they did not have papers. In the end, she accepted neither this injustice nor the narrative that she was undeserving of access to schooling because of her immigration status, and she took steps on her own to further her education.

This book has detailed both the barriers (some of them gendered) that immigrants face in accessing services in the United States and the pipelines to services based on the conditions they have to meet in order to access the safety net. Their strategies for navigating a conditional safety net are crucial to this research, but equally important are immigrants' internal narratives as they navigate an exclusive system. This chapter illustrates respondents pushing back against some of the negative public discourse around Latinx immigrants, including its gendered components, and thus destabilizing larger ideas about who deserves access to services as they question some of the logic that underlies conditional care and reinforce other narratives of deservingness.

Respondents often presented unsolicited narratives that ran counter to the negative public discourse they felt was directed against them. In response to my questions about their experiences accessing services, their interpretations of their immigration status and its impact on them, and their general plans and hopes for the future, one-fifth of the respondents used one or a combination of frames to resist these stigmatizing narratives. That these counternarratives were unsolicited suggests that, despite facing multiple forms of exclusion and exploitation, many respondents resisted internalizing the negative status imposed on them by the narrative of conditional care. Immigrants must contend with the structures of a conditional care system and create strategies to navigate conditional access to services, but they do not necessarily accept the logic of this system. In fact, this chapter demonstrates immigrants' resistance to parts of this logic.

COUNTERNARRATIVES IN RESPONSE TO STIGMATIZATION

By analyzing the discourse of the subset of respondents who directly resisted anti-Latinx immigrant discourse, I found that respondents used at least one of four frames to counter the idea that immigration status is a valid indicator of "illegality" and of moral deservingness of access to services. They demonstrated that far from behaving illegally, they did not break the law (legality frame); they contrasted their strong work ethic to that of the native-born (work frame);

they cast the immigration system that separated families and limited their job opportunities as unjust (injustice frame); and they delegitimized the importance of papers by insisting on their equal self-worth and moral worth relative to others, regardless of their immigration status (equality frame). These frames were gendered in relation to their labor, both in the job market and domestically. I found that the men's positioning of themselves as laborers and the women's positioning of themselves as mothers influenced the frames they used and the actions they took to resist stigmatization and exploitation.

These findings complement the literature on the management of stigma by adding what has been less explored thus far: the perspectives of undocumented immigrants. The analysis here also brings a different lens to the literature, which has traditionally focused on the intentional framings and rearticulations used in broader immigrant rights movements to create the strongest resonance with non-activist individuals. Furthermore, these findings complicate the work on legal consciousness by illustrating that fear, even though it is real and prevalent among first-generation immigrants, does not negate their feelings of self-worth and pride in the broader contribution they make to the United States.[1] Within the perspectives of undocumented immigrants can be found seeds of resistance to the current narrative of deservingness based on immigration status.

By understanding the frames used by non-activist, undocumented immigrants to confront their stigmatization, immigrant rights activists engaged in political mobilization can create a stronger platform that resonates with a broader base, and policymakers can better understand immigrants' own claims countering their exclusion from services based on their immigration status.

"I'm More Legal than the Legal Ones, No?"— Legality as a Counternarrative to Criminalization

Juan was by far one of the boldest respondents in the study, although I didn't expect him to be possessed of such sharp charm and wit when he first came into the day labor center for our interview. He sat by himself, hunched in a chair in the front of the computer area, wearing an orange camouflage hoodie and paint-crusted jeans. As the interview began, he quickly switched from topic to topic, but it soon became unmistakable that Juan was strongly committed to hard work.

He was accustomed to working from a young age, having worked in the fields of his small town along with his family. When work was hard to come by and his mother became ill, Juan made the trip across the border to join his nephews, who had already been working in the construction industry in Concord. Although he was apprehended at the border several times, he kept coming back; at the time of the interview, he had been living continuously in the United States with his sister for over ten years. After battling alcoholism for the better part of the past fifteen years, Juan was now five years sober. His pride in his work, he felt, set him apart from others. After the growing pains of starting out in construction work, he said, his work got better and better over time: "All of the jobs that I do, I don't do them badly—my employers say it's the best."

Even though Juan had earned the respect of his employers, some coworkers still directed racial slurs at him and alluded to his "illegality." When I asked Juan if the racial slurs bothered him, he answered, "No. I'm human just like anyone else. There are some people that get depressed. . . . I don't get depressed. *I'm not from here*, I say" (emphasis added). Although Juan had been living in the United States for over a decade, he still invoked his foreignness as he spoke nonchalantly about people belittling him. That he had been othered made the following statement all the more surprising:

> If I'm legal, illegal, life is the same. They give me work; they give me an opportunity to make money. As long as I have the chance to do that, why would I want to be legal? [Employers] see that I do a good job, and that I respect their things and don't take anything. . . . I'm more legal than the legal ones, no?

Juan simultaneously questioned the importance of papers and challenged the broad claims made by those papers. His lack of papers was supposed to make him "illegal," but what really shaped his legality, he argued, were his actions. Expanding on that idea, Juan said that he had noticed that people with papers were more likely to take things from their employers or to not work as hard. He drew a moral boundary between himself and people deemed "legal" to show that, despite being called "illegal," that label misrepresented his actions.

Juan was one of several respondents who used the frame of legality to combat some of the stigma directed against immigrants and the rhetoric about them as lawbreakers. By using the legality frame to rightly expose the term "illegal" as a misnomer, these respondents were asserting: *I am a fully law-abiding resident.*

Take the example of Pablo, a forty-six-year-old construction worker and father of three who came to the United States for better economic opportunities. I asked Pablo how being undocumented had affected him socially. His response highlighted his economic contribution and law-abiding behavior in paying taxes:

> There are people who are racist and view you as Hispanic and say you don't have papers. That you live off what they pay in taxes. If they knew that I pay more in taxes [because I don't have papers]—I have an ITIN [individual taxpayer identification number], and they don't give me deductions because when I file my taxes, I have to deduct for everything I've earned.

The ITIN allows individuals to pay taxes without having a Social Security number. Even though people with an ITIN pay taxes, they cannot receive Social Security benefits or qualify for the Earned Income Tax Credit (EITC) in most states. The EITC is probably the deduction to which Pablo was referring.[2]

Although men were generally more likely than women to evoke the legality frame to resist anti-immigrant narratives, women did use this frame as well. For instance, I asked Marisol, the talkative working mother of two, whether she was afraid of deportation, and she made use of this frame in her response: "I have been driving for six years, and I haven't been stopped by police. . . . I don't have debts anywhere; I don't owe money anywhere. Since I've started working . . . I've been paying my taxes. I don't see how they would harm me because I don't have any bad record, no crimes, no robberies, no nothing." Other respondents similarly argued that because they worked, paid taxes, and abided by all the laws, they were not suitable candidates for deportation. Although not all respondents challenged the laws that made them subject to deportation in the first place, they did invoke their law-abiding behavior to explain why they deserved to be in the United States.

Immigrants' use of the legality frame directly challenged the rhetoric of immigrants as "rapists," "drug dealers," and "bad hombres" by asserting that they were fully law-abiding individuals.[3] Their economic contribution by paying taxes was important, but most important, they emphasized, was their commitment to the rule of law, despite depictions of them by media outlets and others as "illegal." This framing questions immigration status as an indicator of moral deservingness—an underlying principle of the current conditional safety net—and at the same time it reinforces the importance of law-abiding behavior as an indicator of moral deservingness, to the possible detriment of those with a criminal record who are in need of services. A similar partial resistance to a logic of deservingness shows up in the framing around work.

"They're Not Going to Kick Us Out Because They Need Us": The Work Narrative as a Boundary-Making Strategy and a Critique of the System

In addition to emphasizing their law-abiding behavior in the face of stigma, undocumented respondents in this study also invoked their work ethic to describe their contributions and self-worth. This frame could be deployed to claim status as a "good" and hardworking immigrant in ways that reinforced anti-Blackness and notions of deservingness, or it could be deployed as a deeper critique of the system of exploitative immigrant labor in the United States.

Some discussed the boundary-making frame of hard work as what set them apart from others. Sociologists have extensively studied such ethnic boundary-making and delineated the ways in which ethnic boundaries are continually constructed, reinforced, and sometimes challenged by individuals and institutions. Although those processes share some commonalities, the types of boundaries drawn, reinforced, or challenged can vary by culture and location.[4] For example, racial boundaries are more outwardly pronounced in the United States, but religious boundaries are more prominent in places like the Middle East and Southeast Asia. In this study, some respondents implicitly set themselves apart from native-born racial minorities. It is important to bear in mind that such anti-Black discourse among respondents, whether explicit or implicit, perpetuates negative racial stereotypes that also harm Latinx immigrants. As discussed in the introduction, much of the stigmatization of aid and many of the narratives of deservingness and value judgments that underlie the conditional safety net were formed around anti-Blackness and then weaponized against other racialized groups. Thus, some boundary-making behavior may elevate respondents' self-worth, but at the expense of others, as shown in Isabel's narrative.

Isabel was a forty-three-year-old mother of three adult children and a grandmother of one. Growing up, she had moved from one place to another in Mexico as her widowed mother took care of her and her five sisters. Isabel was able to complete middle school, and in high school she met her soon-to-be husband. They had three children, and after several years of taking care of them in Mexico, Isabel made the trip to Concord. She had spent three years saving up money for her daughter's fifteenth birthday celebration, or *quinceñera*, in Mexico. Isabel was able to return for her daughter's *quinceñera*, but several months later she and her husband decided that it would be best for all three children to come to the United States with her.[5]

Isabel worked multiple jobs cleaning houses, while her husband worked in landscaping. They had divorced two years earlier, and because she had to find and pay for a place of her own, her financial situation worsened. She was able to find a small studio apartment next to a big house in Antioch, and she now worked multiple jobs to make ends meet. Apart from cleaning houses throughout the week, Isabel took care of an elderly woman in the evenings in another suburb. She was frustrated with her limited job options as an undocumented individual:

> There are some people who are bothered because they say that we come here and take away jobs. But if you notice, how many people are out there in the street, under the bridge, asking for money, and they have papers. And a Mexican, for as old as they may be, they're still there [working]. Even if it's picking up the recycling, they're still making money.

Like Juan, Isabel drew a boundary to highlight the work ethic of Mexican immigrants, but she did so by contrasting the work ethic of Mexican immigrants to that of native-born individuals "asking for money." Her boundary-making strategy stigmatized those facing homelessness and poverty and implicitly perpetuated the negative racial stereotype of the Black "welfare queen" who is falsely represented as too "lazy" to work.[6] Other studies have found that some immigrants internalize the false binary of "good" and "bad" immigrants to elevate their own worth as "good" immigrants.[7]

While Isabel's boundary-making discourse perpetuated negative racial stereotypes, it also reflected her deep frustration with the immigration laws. She was clearly aching to work, but her immigration status prevented her from pursuing formal employment. Her frustration became more evident at the end of our interview when Isabel asked me to help her fill out a job application in English.

I started going through the paperwork, translating a few sentences into Spanish for her, and filling it out. It was simple enough to do this until I reached the employer verification section, which included an employer e-verify form stating that her information would be checked with the Department of Justice. We left the e-verify paper blank and provided only some information for the fingerprinting section. I was surprised by how many questions there were on the application about being a U.S. citizen or a lawful resident, and I wondered if Isabel would get the job. I was hesitant about asking her if her contacts who worked there had papers and noticed that she was reluctant to name them as contacts. I grew concerned and uncomfortable as I realized that I was personally running up against the limits imposed by her immigration status.

Like Isabel, Mario also evoked the work frame, but not as a boundary-making strategy to distinguish immigrants as hard workers. Mario evoked the work frame to call out the way the immigration system is set up to exploit labor in the United States. Mario, a forty-five-year-old construction worker and father of two grown adult children in Mexico, had been living in Concord for the past fifteen years. He came from a nine-person household and made his first trip to the United States to help support them. When Mario returned to Mexico, he started his own family. The purpose of his subsequent trip to the United States was to support his wife, who had fallen ill, and to pay their two children's educational expenses. He started working as a day laborer, finding work on street corners and living in crowded housing with other men. But over time he had been able to find stable employment with a small contractor, and he was now able to live on his own.

Describing himself as a solitary man, Mario said that it had been ten years since he last saw his family. When asked how his legal situation affected his life, he commented on U.S. immigration laws and systems of exploitation:

> Those of us who come as immigrants are an unfortunate necessity here. . . . [A] lot of people say that they don't want us . . . but in reality, we're the ones that do the work. . . . And even though they may say that they're going to kick us out, they're not going to kick us out because they need us . . . and they'll always need us.

This framing highlighted the paradox and hypocrisy of a broken immigration system. Even though Americans cast "illegal immigration" as a problem, Mario argued, the national economy is dependent on the exploitation of undocumented workers. He rearticulated the script of undocumented immigrants taking away others' jobs, but flipped it by pointing out that the jobs taken by immigrants are the ones nobody else wants—the labor of immigrants is a critical part of the U.S. economy.

Like Isabel, Mario used the collective "we" to refer to undocumented immigrants. He described his own struggle as bound up with the struggles of others within a broader, structurally broken system. Both men and women in the study used this framing and narrative, but men did so slightly more often. The women were far more likely to frame the immigration system as an injustice to them and their families. These examples show the difference between, on the one hand, claiming to be a hard worker as a way to stigmatize others who are not perceived as equally hardworking, and therefore as equally deserving, and on the other hand, claiming to be a hard worker in a deeper critique of U.S. dependence on a system of exploitative labor.

"We Give the Best to the Country, but the Country Is Not Ready to Give the Best to Us": Viewing the Immigration System through the Injustice Narrative

We saw in this chapter's opening vignette that Magdalena viewed being prevented by her immigration status from taking community college courses to further her college education as an injustice. The theme of injustice was more broadly invoked by the women in the study, especially in their descriptions of how a broken immigration system had harmed them and their families. Many mothers worried about their children being made fun of for being born in a different country and hence accused of being "illegal," or they lamented their inability to take their children to other states for fear of being caught. When I asked Magdalena about how her immigration status affected her, she said:

> It's different. You can't go out for fun, you can't go on vacation. . . . No, here there is always fear, so we have to stay in the city, and what can we do? The children aren't at fault. . . . They need to live and feel normal. I mean, they don't have to feel less than other people because [their parents] made the decision to come here. It was me, not them.

Pati, the mother of three we met earlier, similarly felt that the current immigration system is set up against undocumented immigrants, and she worried endlessly about its effect on her oldest daughter, who was born in Mexico and was also undocumented upon coming to the United States. As her daughter grew up, Pati advised her to not mention where she was from; if anybody asked her, Pati instructed her, she was to say that she was born in Oakland. Pati had heard of children making fun of other children for being "illegal," and she didn't want her daughter to be bullied because of her status.

At the time of the interview, Pati was feeling hopeful: her daughter had become a DACA recipient and was going to college.[8] Overall, however, Pati felt stressed from the difficulty of paying rent, and being unable to access rental assistance programs because of her immigration status only added to the stress:

> In the years that my husband barely had work, it was really difficult to [have food to] eat, to pay the rent, it was almost impossible. It didn't help that we didn't have access to rental aid. . . . [My immigration status] is a big barrier. We give the best to the country, but the country is not ready to give the best to us. Maybe one day. We must keep trying and try to be the best we can be.

Pati explicitly called out the immigration system's negative impact on her and her family. As undocumented immigrants, she pointed out, they contributed to the country, giving it their best, but the country, unjustly, did not provide reciprocal support to undocumented communities, even though they were in need of it.

Pati later said, "Even though I was born in Mexico, I appreciate and respect what I have received here, and I respect everyone here. The family separation that the immigration raids create greatly affect the country's progress. The best values come from the family, and that is the best for the country." In this statement, Pati revealed how nonsensical the immigration raids are. Like many immigrants, she respected everybody and instilled that value in her children. What sense did it make for immigration laws to separate her family when she was raising her children to be respectful, kind citizens?

Although women were more apt to describe the immigration system as unjust, men also saw the injustice of the immigration system and questioned what was gained from immigration raids. Ronaldo, whom we met in the last chapter, had heard about people being deported who were not criminals, and he felt that they did not deserve to be separated from their families. Those raids, he said, were "completely unjust. . . . They came to find one person . . . and they took away the whole family. . . . They're not delinquents. They're citizens that work. They're earning an honest living. They have their own apartment; they pay rent; they're not parasites. . . . They're people that, that fight." Although this frame may play into the frame of the "good" immigrant, versus the parasitic or delinquent immigrant, it leaves open the possibility for a deeper critique of an exploitative and unjust immigration system. Counter to a narrative that frames immigrants as lawbreakers by definition, Ronaldo named the system of deportation itself as unjust. Other men similarly lamented the raids that broke apart families and worried to some extent about being separated from their own families in the United States.

"I Only Have Toilet Paper!": Using Humor and Equality Narratives to Challenge Stigma

Some respondents questioned the intentions and consequences of the law by taking it a step further: they devalued and mocked the terminology and logic of "having papers." Although there were many somber moments during the interviews for this research, there were also some moments interrupted by humor and lightness. One of the most memorable such moments came from Estanislao, a thirty-eight-year-old father of three who came to the United States to better support his three children, who still lived in Guatemala.

Despite a rocky start in the United States while he stayed with an unsupportive family member in Los Angeles, Estanislao had now forged his own path in Oakland with the help of another family member and was working odd jobs in construction to support himself and send money home to his children. He was undocumented and had no steady income from his job as a day laborer, but he maintained a chipper, almost jovial, attitude throughout the interview. For instance, when I asked Estanislao if the topic of immigration status ever came up in conversations with his friends, he responded, "Sometimes my *compas* (friends) will ask me, 'Do you have papers?' 'No,' I say, 'I only have toilet paper!' " followed by a hearty laugh.

Juan, mentioned in the beginning of the chapter, said that when others used derogatory terms like "wetback," he would respond that he had just showered that morning. Through his use of humor, Juan delegitimized the importance attached to whether a person had papers or not and directly confronted and challenged derogatory terms.

In discussing why they did not see themselves as different from people with papers, respondents used the equality frame in ways similar to others' use of the injustice frame. Some insisted that, like anyone else, they had a right to fair wages. They either emphasized the equality of all people or asserted that, as long as they had work, their immigration status should not make them any different from others. Typical remarks were along the lines of, "With documents or without documents, I have value," or, "Well, for me, not having papers or having papers is the same, it doesn't make me any better or worse [than others]." Unlike the frame of challenging immigration laws, the equality frame focuses on challenging the stigma attached to individuals' immigration status by evoking notions of equal individual self-worth.

REFUSING CONDITIONS OF EXCLUSION

Respondents not only developed counternarrative frames to resist anti-immigrant narratives but also refused, through their actions, to accede to exclusions. Magdalena, for instance, circumvented exclusionary laws by finding workarounds that would allow her to pursue higher education. For Rosario, simply telling others about the resources available to low-income individuals and the undocumented community was a way to build collective knowledge and push back against a system of exclusions and structural violence. She had recently discovered a Facebook group where people from different neighborhoods, blocks, and towns could showcase their businesses and post announcements about, for example, upcoming community events. The group was run by Spanish speakers, and she saw that several people were using this resource and asking for information on affordable clinics. Rosario quickly posted about the free clinic she went to, and she also said that anybody who had a question about services could dial the number 2-1-1—a bit of information she had learned from a nonprofit organization she was involved in. She said that it had felt "necessary" to share the information because, when she herself was new to the community, "I didn't know where to go." Beyond posting information about free clinics and other services and resources, Rosario had also helped her neighbor secure Section 8 housing, even though she herself wasn't eligible for it. Rosario in many ways was "paying it forward" while also pushing back against laws that were exclusionary toward immigrants by serving as a guiding figure for other people.

Work and Refusal

While Rosario, Magdalena, and many others refused to acquiesce to exclusionary policies toward immigrants by seeking out services and accruing resources, others talked more directly about resisting oppressive structures in the workplace. Even when such forms of resistance were met with pushback, as often happened, these respondents insisted on fair treatment and wages.

A case in point was Mayra, a fifty-four-year-old mother of three grown children. A former dry cleaning worker and caregiver, Mayra had spent the past eighteen years in the United States. When I asked about the impact on her life of her immigration status, she responded, "A lot of people say, 'You have to adapt to whatever is given to you.' For example, a job that pays you [low wages] because one doesn't have a [Social Security number]. They say, 'You have to put up with it.' I had a job ironing at a dry cleaner, and I had to get out of there." Besides paying her low wages without overtime, the dry cleaner owners had berated her for looking at the clock during work. Mayra told them that she simply looked at the clock so she could know the time, but the owners weren't having it. They called her stupid and told her to leave the building. As she described this episode, Mayra defiantly asserted the ridiculousness of the accusation.

She did not return to work at the dry cleaner after that incident and instead began taking care of children, which she had now done for the last several years. In this work as well, she challenged her exploitation. Her employers would pay her only $20 to $25 for taking care of their children for approximately ten hours. Taking care of multiple children was not easy; she had to change their diapers, feed them, and engage them in playtime while keeping them safe from harm. One of her friends who also took care of children told her, "You are giving away your work. They pay me $110 a day. I go to my employer's home, but the only thing I do is take care of one baby." Taking her friend's advice into account, Mayra raised her price to $30 to $35 a day. When her employers resisted, she stopped taking care of their children. Her three grown children had enough money to support her, so after devoting a majority of her life to taking care of others, Mayra decided to focus on herself instead. Besides unionization and direct confrontation, refusing to participate in unfair treatment can also be a way of resisting exploitative working conditions.

Enrique was a forty-year-old restaurant and retail worker with a young daughter in the United States. His remarks at the end of the interview, when I asked him if there was anything else he wanted to say about being an immigrant living in the United States, provided another illustration of refusal to accept conditions of hyperexploitation:

I feel like, even myself, [we] illegal immigrants sometimes close opportunities for ourselves. . . . We restrict ourselves by saying, "Oh well, I'm illegal, so I can only work in gardening or construction, or restaurants." Yeah, but we don't ask to see if we can get work in a business that's—bigger, that would [enable us] to use benefits.

Enrique was one of the few undocumented respondents in this study who had a job in the formal labor market and consequently was also one of the few who had full health insurance coverage from his employer. His decision to pursue a job in the formal labor market was his way of showing that the immigration system was not going to dictate the terms of his life in the United States. Although few other respondents had taken the action of seeking work in the formal labor market, Enrique's decision to do so is one more example of immigrants contesting narratives that they do not deserve fair compensation and purposely defying laws meant to exclude them and exploit their labor simply because of their immigration status.

Everyday Refusal

This chapter has shown that undocumented immigrants use the frames of legality, work, injustice, and equality to challenge their stigmatization as "illegal." Respondents in this study refused narratives of their criminality by highlighting their law-abiding behavior, asserting that they were hard workers whose labor was integral to the United States, and eloquently describing the injustices of immigration laws. Some claimed their equality with people with papers, regardless of what others said.

These frames exposed the contradictions and paradoxes of the immigration system, some of which were present in respondents' own answers. Even though the federal government claims to be "kicking undocumented immigrants out," the United States depends on their labor. Despite respondents' claims to equality, they still cast themselves as outsiders given the opportunity to work in an exploitative labor market. Respondents might not have flipped the script entirely, but strong tones of defiance and triumph, despite living in a country that continued to oppress them, could be heard in their voices. They saw the stigmatization and criminalization of everyone of their status, but they refused to let that script wholly define how they saw themselves and how they conceived of their self-worth.

Respondents' narratives and actions mirror the ways in which other marginalized communities defy stigmatizing discourses and oppressive structures. The use of transgressive narratives and actions to counter hegemonic ideals dates back centuries, to when slaves contested their subordinate position with tactics such as foot-dragging, feigning ignorance, sabotaging crops, or even running away. Slaves also created transgressive narratives that explicitly denounced their structural oppression. These so-called hidden transcripts were "discourse that takes place 'offstage,' beyond direct observation by powerholders."[9] Hidden transcripts have the power to challenge and contest hegemonic narratives; while providing, at a minimum, a space to vent about structural injustices, they may also sow the seeds for broader collective action.

In his study of peasants and landowners in Malaysia in the 1980s, the political scientist James Scott notes that peasants invoked a worldview that prioritized an individual's morality and work ethic over profit and capital gain—the goals of the wealthy landowning class. In disavowing the moral authority of the dominant class, these Malaysian peasants rejected the symbolic authority of the wealthy landowning class over them.[10]

Decades later, in much the same way, the sociologist Michèle Lamont found that working-class, non-college-educated men in the United States and France used similar moral boundaries to distance themselves from both poor populations (particularly in the United States) and rich populations (in both countries).[11] By emphasizing their strong work ethic and upstanding moral character, working-class men maintained dignity in the face of a changing economy that increasingly marginalized their economic and social position. In a similar fashion, the sociologist Crystal Fleming and her colleagues' interview-based study in the United States found that when confronted with stigmatizing discourse in interpersonal interactions, most African Americans directly challenge others to "teach themselves" about racism. Still, a few reluctantly engage in intentional emotional management in order to contain their anger and emphasize their professional identity so as not to perpetuate negative stereotypes about African Americans as "loud" and "angry."[12] Although these means of refusing narratives and oppressive structures are inspirational and, in many ways, necessary for social change, they also point to the chronic wear and tear on the minds and bodies of those who are societally stigmatized.[13]

The frames used by respondents in this study mirror the frames that have been employed by various immigration social movements through the decades. The frames of hard work, family unity, law abidance, and assimilation were effectively used by early activists in the DREAMer movement and by the organizers of the widespread 2006 immigration marches. Starting in 2010, activists began using more confrontational frames that called out the broken immigration system and contested the notion of "good" or "bad" immigrants. Instead of reinforcing the false notion of individual immigrants as either "good" or "bad," they pointed to the unequal structures that render *every* immigrant "illegal" and further dehumanize and exclude undocumented and mixed-status households through punitive immigration policies.

As we have seen in this chapter, there are some overlaps in immigrants' and activists' frames of legality, work and boundary-making, and injustice; we have also seen that humor and the equality frame are less commonly used and invoked. Notably, humor is visible in undocuqueer activism, which uses comedy to humanize the experiences of undocumented youth.[14] More generally, humor is also used in educational settings as a mode of resistance by immigrant students and their families.[15]

Gendered Narratives

There were also gendered differences among respondents in the frames they used. Women more often used the injustice frame and discussed the effects of immigration policies on their children and their livelihood. In contrast, only men used the equality frame and questioned the importance of papers. These gendered differences mirror those found in past studies, some of which have shown that undocumented women become emboldened to claim their motherhood and redefine citizenship.[16] Others have found that undocumented men emphasize their work ethic as part of their identity and use this to draw a distinction between themselves and native-born U.S. citizens or documented immigrants.[17]

These differences between men and women may reflect their family structures and work atmospheres. I recruited the men in the study from day labor centers, which require that employers provide a dignified working atmosphere and pay at least the minimum wage. These labor centers are also associated with nonprofit organizations that engage in advocacy that members can become involved in, such as participating in the Labor Day march for workers' rights in Oakland. That said, none of the respondents were involved in direct advocacy for workers or immigrants. In fact, the most powerful statements contesting the legitimacy of being required to have papers were made by respondents who had the least at stake in the United States. They did not have families here, and some said that they were not afraid of deportation. Perhaps, having less at stake, they were able to more fearlessly accuse the system of being unjust and more open to adopting new frames to demonstrate their moral worth. Other works in the immigration literature have shown that those who are least "embedded" in systems have a different legal consciousness than those with active bureaucratic or administrative records.[18]

Not all respondents fearlessly sought out social services or filed labor claims in the event of an accident, though not because they thought immigration laws and policies were morally acceptable. The hidden transcripts described in this chapter may not always result in actionable behaviors, but the frames developed by immigrants themselves can resonate with other immigrant populations, especially in appeals to collective action.

The sociologists Irene Bloemraad, Kimberly Voss, and Fabiana Silva conducted a survey of nearly two thousand randomly sampled California residents to compare how using the frames of economic contribution, family unity, and human rights affected people's views on undocumented immigrants having a pathway to citizenship and using public services.[19] Their survey data showed that, while the human rights frame has the most potential for expanding notions of American citizenship and inclusivity, it resonates the least with the public. In addition, the frame of economic contribution, which is commonly used in the immigrant rights movement, does little to sway public opinion on legalization or provision of public services to undocumented immigrants. Instead, family unity was the strongest frame, especially among self-reported conservatives. In a similar study on framing, researchers found that the tactic of using a framing of "opportunity" versus "amnesty" and describing immigrants as "law-abiding" versus "lawbreaking" was more likely to garner support for providing a pathway to citizenship for immigrants.[20] Although it is important that those attempting to pass immigration reform understand which frames appeal most to voters, it is equally, if not more, important to know which frames resonate best with those who are deeply affected by the immigration laws in place—undocumented immigrants themselves. It is also important to be aware of which narrative tactics can serve to gain temporary comparative advantage at the cost of bolstering a system that eventually leads to overall harm, such as designating oneself a hard worker in contrast to those in other marginalized groups or criminalized groups. For example, the temporary increase in sympathy or support for those who always "follow the law" risks dehumanizing or villainizing those who have had contact with the carceral system. It is important not to use these frames in a way that further entrenches carceral institutions and justifies austerity.

Especially in times of federal immigrant exclusion, the seeds of internal resistance have tremendous potential to grow. As discussed further in the next chapter, the push for more humane immigration policies must begin by disrupting both the narrative of the undocumented immigrant as a "criminal" *and* the narrative of the undocumented immigrant as a "victim." Instead, we must focus our energies on the increasingly fragile foundation upon which the national safety net is built. Millions of people, whether undocumented or not, suffer from a bare, thin, and fragmented welfare system because it is a system that prioritizes individual wealth and capital gain over collective well-being.

This book focuses on the consequences of an exclusionary welfare state for Latinx and immigrant populations, but the repercussions of a restrictive and thinning safety net negatively affect us all. The concluding chapter explains why it is in our best interest to implement policies that build a more robust and inclusive safety net for all as well as to reimagine a world in which providing care to people is no longer up for debate.

CHAPTER 6

Conclusion: Moving toward Unconditional Care

This book has sought to answer two questions: How do immigrants navigate a limited and exclusionary safety net in the United States? And what factors impede or facilitate their access to social services? By providing some answers to these questions, this book hopes to offer insights to service providers aiming to create more inclusive access to services, policymakers seeking to create more just institutional practices, and academics working to gain better insight into systems of exclusion and tactics of accessing care.

Through two years of fieldwork and eighty-five interviews with people whose incomes were limited and immigration statuses were liminal, this book has detailed how the safety net conditions the types of services that individuals can (or cannot) receive based on their income, their gendered roles, and their immigration status. These conditions put up legal, linguistic, psychological, and logistical barriers for noncitizens seeking basic services like food assistance and health care. These barriers are more pronounced in suburban spaces, which have limited public transportation and fewer local nonprofit organizations; NPOs that offer linguistically and culturally competent programs are particularly scarce in the suburbs.

To navigate a system of conditional care, people call on their social networks to facilitate their access to services. Undocumented individuals benefit from knowing someone who shares their immigration status and can vouch for services, particularly government programs, and who can reassure them when they sign up for assistance that it is safe to do so. Women in this study often described having a "guiding figure" or trusted confidante who not only informed them about different services but also offered rides to health clinics, nonprofit organizations, and governmental administrative offices to sign up for benefits or receive services.

In contrast, the men in this study had access to fewer social services. Many of the men had left their family in their country of origin; with no children to provide an opening into services, they were largely left out of the safety net, from which those who were undocumented were already largely excluded. They typically sought health care only when they had a medical emergency (many of which were workplace injuries). With no private or public insurance coverage, some of these men had been left with huge medical expenses they could not pay. Those men whose networks informed them about worker centers had a somewhat better experience finding health care. Not only were they connected to employment opportunities at these centers, but they also learned about services they could access, such as federally qualified health centers and county-based programs offering health services.

Respondents used the legality, work, injustice, and inequality frames to counter the negative stereotypes of undocumented and Latinx immigrants that underlie the negative discourses justifying the restriction of resources available to racialized populations. The legality and work frames focused on individual boundary-making and moral claims. The immigrants who drew boundaries between themselves and people born in the United States—particularly Black and Latinx individuals, as well as the unstably housed—ran the risk of negatively stereotyping these populations. In contrast, the justice and equality frames challenged the logic of systematically exclusionary systems that create racial and class hierarchies.

EMPIRICAL AND THEORETICAL CONTRIBUTIONS OF THIS STUDY

The findings of this book have several implications for scholars and practitioners aiming to understand existing barriers to services and to create more equitable access to resources.

Immigration Status and Place Analysis of Safety Net Access

Welfare state scholars commonly focus on how native-born respondents access and navigate public programs.[1] In addition, they almost exclusively focus on the experiences of mothers using cash assistance.[2] Fewer studies examine noncitizens' access to the welfare state, and fewer still look at access for undocumented immigrants.[3] By focusing on how immigration status shapes access to services, I show the importance of bonding ties in creating trust, sharing information, and gaining access to resources. In other words, hearing about an assistance program from somebody who is in a similar position and has already participated in that program fosters a sense of safety in accessing services, particularly from government programs. This book also excavates the gendered terrain of access to social services for men and women of different immigration statuses. The analysis demonstrates how gender and immigration status *intersect* to facilitate or impede an individual's access to public and private aid.[4]

The suburbanization of poverty literature is predominantly a quantitative literature that shows spatial mismatches between service providers and populations in need.[5] By bringing in suburban residents' narratives on accessing social services, this book contributes to that literature by showing that personal networks can mitigate some of the harmful effects of the relative lack of resources in suburban locations. For those who are socially isolated, however, living in a suburban place may worsen the effects of their isolation and reduce their chances of accessing services.

In focusing on immigrant populations, the book also shows how individuals and families cope with legal and linguistic barriers to accessing social services, which may be more pronounced in a suburban space. At the same time, the book underscores the potential silver lining of seeking services in a more constrained resource landscape: where there are fewer organizations, they are more likely to be known to each other, and that familiarity can create opportunities for cohesion and cooperation among organizations as they work toward the same goals.

Conditional Safety

This book bridges the literatures on welfare, geography, and immigration by advancing the concept of "conditional safety." Scholars have begun excavating the intersection and contours of the criminal legal system and the immigration state in what has been termed "crimmigration."[6] This punitive state legally and psychologically restricts the freedoms of noncitizens as they decide whether to drive, go out, or visit family or friends; choose a neighborhood to live in; engage in acts of political activism and mobilization; or apply for and receive services or assistance to meet their basic needs.[7] Fear of family separation, deportation, or other forms of punishment looms large for Latinx immigrants—and probably for other immigrants as well, across all immigration statuses, including U.S. citizens in mixed-status households—and the extent of those fears is largely shaped by local sociopolitical contexts.[8] In my interviews, this fear also included future hypotheticals, such as concern that accessing services in the present would complicate a future pathway to residency or citizenship. This atmosphere of threat can prevent people from seeking out assistance to meet their basic needs, even services for which they would qualify.

Although we use terms like "safety net" (to describe public benefit programs), "sanctuary cities," and "sensitive areas," this research reveals that federal laws, with their accompanying risks and restrictions, permeate ostensibly "safe" spaces.[9] Respondents in this study remained rightfully wary of sharing information with public institutions such as schools, hospitals, and clinics. These institutions have cooperated with ICE in the past, and breaches of this policy only increased during the Trump administration.[10] The sanctity of such spaces simply cannot be taken for granted.

Policies regarding public benefits for noncitizen populations are always prone to change, and federal policies governing noncitizens' access to public programs have only become more stringent in the past five decades.[11] State and local actors create protections for their residents, but these protections are always limited. Any form of protection for undocumented and noncitizen populations from surveillance and deportation is always conditional. Even when one administration advances immigrant protections at the federal level, they can be vetoed or weakened in the next.

Gendered Knowledge-Sharing

This study has shown how structure and culture work together to facilitate or impede relations with the state. Structurally, the presence of public programs for pregnant persons or parents with young children creates a gendered condition for what some scholars fittingly describe as the left, or "maternal," side of the state. This structure is then reinforced by a culture of information-sharing in women's networks, ensuring that many of those eligible will gain access to these programs. By contrast, the restriction of any such programs for men interacts with a culture of hegemonic masculinity to make immigrant men's access to services much more limited. The fact that the conditions of access to care are narrow for noncitizens, even narrower for undocumented populations, and narrowest of all for undocumented single men is alarming given men's overall lower health indicators and higher risk of surveillance and deportation.[12]

Administrative Burden

The complex conditions needed to access safety net programs have been described by scholars as administrative burdens. Administrative burdens are composed of the learning cost to become informed about programs, the psychological cost of navigating such programs, and the compliance cost of fulfilling the requirements to continue participation in them.[13] The concept of conditional care expands the concept of administrative burden by focusing on the logic that undergirds the conditions that shape not only the ease of accessing services but also the possibility of being eligible for them in the first place. A "No Wrong Door" motto has taken hold as a model for more inclusive social service provision, the idea being to give clients multiple entrances into programs, like multiple doors into a building. Although this approach is a step forward, the concept of conditional access focuses on understanding not just the existing doors but who is allowed to walk through them.

THE LIMITATIONS OF THIS RESEARCH

This book has focused on gendered social networks as facilitators of access to services and resources rather than the exploitation that individuals sometimes face upon arrival in the United States. Such exploitation can hinder immigrants' access to crucial resources and services, and some respondents in this study reported having had exploitative experiences. They described being subject to abuse in their families and informal networks as well as in the workplace, often at the hands of coethnic employers or connections, as documented in some studies.[14] Some had thought there was someone they could connect to for a job or housing, but the connection fell through. Others were told by family members not to apply for services, or they were used by some in their informal networks for childcare and cooking. Some even had their savings stolen. As Menjívar argues, the networks that migrants enter into are also facing resource constraints that shape the support they are able and willing to offer to others.[15] Moreover, in more isolated geographical areas, migrants are at greater risk of being exploited by their personal or coethnic networks.[16] That said, the findings of this study overwhelmingly pointed to social networks as a main vehicle for information and logistical support.

Because everyone that I spoke to in this study was a Latinx immigrant, the ways in which networks can serve as vehicles of information and the types of information that they can provide can vary for different immigrant networks. For example, Esther Cho's study of undocumented Asian and Latinx immigrants found that Asian immigrants were connected to a wider variety of labor markets, owing to the more diverse nature of their networks.[17] That said, immigrant populations who speak a language other than Spanish may face more linguistic or different sets of cultural barriers to participating in public benefits programs, which could impact their participation rates.[18] Future research should be devoted to the mechanisms that shape how non-Latinx immigrant populations navigate the safety net and how this is impacted by immigration status.[19]

About 60 percent of the respondents I spoke to were recruited from non-profit organizations, such as food pantries, community-based centers, day labor centers, and childcare centers. Their experiences represent the best-case scenarios of people who eventually connected to services, so an understanding of the experiences of people who do not end up becoming connected to services may be underdeveloped. That said, among the fully 40 percent of the sample recruited from churches, flea markets, and referrals, the mechanisms for connecting to care remained the same for women; for men, I found that those who were not connected to day labor centers were even less likely to be connected to any form of care, except in medical emergencies.

It should also be noted that the study was based in a politically progressive state and in cities with more pro-immigrant policies and programs in place to buffer the federally exclusive system. In more restrictive states or local political contexts, where there is less political impetus to provide resources for immigrant communities, the ability to access social services looks even bleaker, as has been indicated by studies in those settings.[20] There may be fewer coethnic networks through which to share information, or those very networks may be more exploitative in a less immigrant-friendly place. Moreover, the landscape of social service organizations, especially those that offer culturally focused care, may be sparser. In places with heavier police surveillance or more internal border checkpoints, the risk of traveling for care is even greater—a risk that can be heightened for men who are more likely to be targeted for deportation.[21] Moreover, this research does not cover the experiences of those in more rural contexts, the study of which has been undertaken by other immigration scholars.[22] Given the federal policy constraints that limit access to care, however, and even with relatively open conditions to care in the Bay Area, the insights here concerning how immigrants are constrained from access to care remain relevant regardless of geographic location.

All the respondents in this study were cisgender, and all of them reported being in a heterosexual relationship. This research thus does not capture the wide variety of experiences along the gender and sexuality spectrums that are likely to impact social networks, available resources, and the resource-seeking process. I was able to focus the study on only a few points of comparison: gender, immigration status, and place. Future studies could do comparative analyses among LGBTQIA+ populations and between Indigenous and non-Indigenous populations, as well as between respondents of different countries of origin.[23]

At the time of this study, the temporary protected status of individuals from El Salvador was not in question; however, it came into question in 2018 and became yet another factor in people's eligibility for programs and their decisions about whether to participate in them. Finally, all the interviews for this study were conducted before the Trump administration. Prior to 2016, many individuals had noted the gains made on behalf of immigrants in the previous year, including DACA at the federal level and AB 60 in California. The latter allowed California residents to receive a driver's license regardless of their immigration status—a move that vastly increased mobility and reduced fear of deportation in people's everyday lives.

THE POLICY IMPLICATIONS OF THIS RESEARCH
Inclusive Safety Net Policies

California is one of the most politically progressive states—if not *the* most politically progressive—when it comes to expanding the safety net. In 2020, the state expanded Medi-Cal eligibility to individuals under the age of twenty-six who meet the criteria for Medi-Cal, regardless of their immigration status. In 2021, California was one of the first states to expand Earned Income Tax Credit eligibility to those who file their taxes with an ITIN.[24] And in May 2022, California expanded Medi-Cal access to people age fifty and older whose immigration status previously excluded them from public health coverage. It is estimated that this expansion will impact approximately 185,000 people who have had to rely on a patchwork of FQHCs and free medical clinics to have their medical needs met as they age—or who have received no care at all.[25] In May 2022, Medi-Cal expanded access to all eligible individuals, regardless of their immigration status; this will take effect by January 1, 2024.[26] This was after a decade of research and advocacy efforts by a coalition of over one hundred organizations that pushed for more inclusive health care access under the campaign of Health4All.

At a more local level, programs like Healthy SF, Healthy Families in LA, and even the HealthPAC program in Alameda County have pushed for primary care services to be more inclusive and readily available to those in need. Though less expansive in scope, the Contra Costa Cares program, with strong and consistent local mobilization, could be a starting point for expanding services.[27] Health care advocates achieved one of their greatest successes in 2015 when California expanded Medi-Cal access to all minors, regardless of their immigration status.

This study showed that state interventions and policies created the widest form of access for women. Residents need to keep pushing their representatives for these public programs so that private organizations can focus less on providing medical resources themselves and more on connecting the right populations to needed public services.[28] Yes, there is a chance that this information could be negatively used by the federal government, but having these programs in place would give individuals and families the option of deciding for themselves whether they will apply.

Apart from expanding access to social services, numerous policies could be enacted to mitigate the harmful effects of legal violence against legally liminal populations. For instance, municipal IDs could be created for city residents, enabling everyone to have a valid form of identification to use to open bank accounts or verify their identity at schools, hospitals, workplaces, and other institutions that typically ask for formal identification.[29] Another option would be to make all local residents, regardless of their immigration status, eligible to apply for a driver's license, which would give undocumented individuals more peace of mind when they drive. They would also be able to avoid costly citations (and possible car impoundments) for driving without a license. Such a policy has been passed in California, and respondents in this study reported that the new policy reduced the chronic stress they had felt from driving without a license.

Worker centers provide a place for individuals to seek employment at fair wages and to report abusive behavior or exploitation by employers. Many of these centers are funded by grants from local foundations and business sponsors; creating sustainable public sources of funding for these centers could go a long way toward extending their reach.[30] In the absence of public health coverage for most undocumented individuals, FQHCs and other medical clinics have been a significant source of health care for this population. Expanding funding for these clinics and developing ways to streamline access to their services, particularly mental health services, could go a long way toward ensuring that these critical services are accessible to those most in need. Moreover, policymakers could propose targeted investments for suburban and rural community-based organizations to provide resources for establishing multilingual and culturally competent care for immigrant or other Black, Indigenous, and other People of Color (BIPOC) populations.

In addition to worker centers, a key set of organizational institutions that I did not explore in this book are the services and resources offered by consulates. The Mexican consulate played a pivotal role in coordinating outreach efforts and providing legal aid and financial support for Mexican nationals applying to the DACA program; other scholarship has noted that Mexican and other Latin American consulates have bolstered a wide range of services in New York and California. Specifically related to health care, the Ventanilla de Salud ("Health Window") program was established by the Mexican consulate to eliminate barriers to health care for Mexican nationals living in the United States. One of the main informational outreach efforts is the Binational Health Week, which was inaugurated in 2001 by the Health Initiative of the Americas at the University of California–Berkeley. At this annual event, consular agencies from Latin American countries, NPOs, churches, and hometown organizations provide educational workshops, information, and health services for Latin American immigrant communities across the nation. Although these initiatives and programs were not mentioned by respondents in this research, funding for these initiatives should not be overlooked.[31] The same can be said for organizations, such as Mission Asset Fund, that formalize existing community structures, like *tandas* (lending circles), to help build credit for populations that may not have access to formal credit systems in the United States. Most recently, Mission Asset Fund launched a cash aid program to help individuals and families that were financially impacted by the COVID-19 pandemic.[32] An important element of all the efforts and policies named here is the energy and resources dedicated to research and evaluation to determine the most effective and impactful best practices for improving health outcomes.

Beyond creating more inclusive policies for immigrant populations, there is an opportunity to create fewer conditions of access to care for people who have been excluded because of their criminal record, gender identity, sexual orientation, or disability or for those who have been discriminated against based on their race. Scholars have already broken ground on developing frameworks for defamilizing the welfare state and enabling labor force participation by reducing the need for caregiving by the family.[33] Taking it one step further, some scholars have outlined ways to degender the welfare state so as to facilitate the caregiving responsibilities of anyone, regardless of their gender. The avenues to an inclusive safety net are widely diverse; this book touches on only a portion of what makes access to care conditional.

Broader Immigration Reform

The exclusion of individuals from services based on their immigration status would be alleviated if immigration status was not a form of exclusion in the first place. The passage of DACA benefited undocumented parents as well as their children, DACA's beneficiaries. The DACA program has benefited thousands of families, but it is narrow in the scope of who is eligible and has been criticized for feeding into dangerous narratives of deservingness by including only those who are deemed to have good "moral character."[34] Preserving this program but, more importantly, expanding eligibility for a pathway to U.S. citizenship through broader immigration reform, such as amnesty, would allow millions of individuals to envision greater upward financial and social mobility in their future. At a minimum, considering more flexible or open policies around work-based permits or visas could make it easier for immigrants to contribute to the formal economy while also allowing for more circular patterns of migration that allow people to live transnational lives and maintain connections with communities in multiple places.

Developing and Reinforcing Inclusive Rights-Based Framing

In efforts to pass more inclusive safety net policies, framing matters.[35] In a recent public meeting in Concord, a Contra Costa County representative stood in front of a crowded room and stated her support for expanding health services for immigrant populations. In her call to mobilize for such reform, she suggested that people convince their friends and neighbors that expanding health care access is a public health issue, since not providing medical care can lead to the spread of communicable disease. Acknowledging that this perspective was "selfish," she said that she was proposing expanding health care access as a way to reach across the aisle.

Although her intentions were well meaning, her suggested justification for expanding health care services, by invoking stereotypes of immigrants as "dirty," did little to humanize immigrant populations.[36] All of us, including policymakers and politicians, must be mindful of the language we use to frame and describe marginalized populations so as to avoid contributing to racialized discourses and negative stereotypes that dehumanize and otherize millions of people and justify excluding them from basic services to meet their needs.

Improving Labor Conditions and Standards

Although access to services and the safety net is important, I would be remiss if I did not address the larger structural conditions that make immigrant populations vulnerable in the first place. Their vulnerability is maintained through unjust immigration laws, exploitative labor markets, and a global capitalist state that values profit over individual health and human rights. My interviews revealed that one of the biggest sources of anxiety for many respondents was their financial instability from working in unpredictable, low-wage jobs. This worry was only worsened by rising costs of living from soaring rent prices and neighborhood gentrification. Policy initiatives that would allow undocumented University of California students to be eligible for work-study programs to help pay for their tuition, such as Opportunity for All, are one step toward reducing the barriers to employment that affect people's well-being.[37]

Current labor standards do not provide much economic security even for people in the formal workforce; health is also impaired as minimum wages fall well below current standards for a living wage, and limited sick days, vacation days, parental leave, and other worker protections leave workers with little room for meeting their financial and health needs.[38] These issues affect many California residents across racial and ethnic lines. Finding ways to work with and across populations experiencing intersecting forms of marginalization creates perhaps the most powerful form of solidarity to advocate for a system that promotes inclusive care. At an individual level, a wide set of actions can be taken to work toward a more inclusive safety net: jumpstarting, financially supporting, or becoming involved in advocacy campaigns to open up access to social services or employment for historically and presently excluded populations (such as undocumented populations) from the safety net; hiring individuals from worker centers or other worker cooperatives who are guaranteed a living wage in their jobs; or simply reframing conversations with others not only to avoid a logic of deservingness of various forms of support and care but also to question why that logic exists. Although seemingly small, such actions can have ripple effects and are necessary if change is to be achieved on a larger scale.

Creating a Universal Safety Net

Many of the policy suggestions detailed earlier are short- or medium-term efforts that could be pursued at this moment. The reality, however, is that transforming a conditional safety net into a universal one will be a long journey. Beyond expanding the safety net to people regardless of their immigration status, the United States needs to reexamine the current criteria used to determine eligibility for public benefits—one of the most critical being the way the poverty threshold is determined. Using a poverty threshold from the 1960s—when housing costs were expected to amount to only one-third of people's living expenses—ignores the reality of today's housing costs in California and other coastal states that have been dealing with long-standing housing crises. Exploring the possibility of establishing programs like universal basic income (UBI) or restitutive policies at a local level could lay the groundwork for expanding such policies on a larger scale.[39]

The purpose of sociology is to expose the nuances of what some may consider obvious truths to fully understand origins, implications, and fissures. The safety net in the United States, from its history through the present, assumes a logic of guilty until proven innocent. A preoccupation with people "taking advantage" of programs has dominated the national narrative on welfare rather than a preoccupation with people not having the proper resources to survive and thrive. If we continue to uphold a narrative that reinforces the need to "earn" care, the default will be not caring for ourselves or for others. This uncaring logic harms us all. This book is not the first to make this argument, but in doing so it has detailed an empirical case study of how this logic fails millions of individuals and families residing in the United States.

When social policies are created by those who are not directly impacted by them, the result is austerity, surveillance, and othering. Although this book offers some suggestions on constructing a universal social safety net, I urge readers to reimagine what inclusive welfare could be by looking beyond this book and toward the individuals, communities, and institutions that are presently navigating the social safety net and know it best. It is my hope that in furthering an understanding of the contours, contradictions, and avenues, both closed and open, of access to public services and resources, this book will contribute to long-standing and current efforts to reenvision and work toward a safety net that provides meaningful support to everyone in need of resources and care.

EPILOGUE

The last interview for this book took place the day Donald Trump was elected to the presidency. Leading up to the election, several respondents mentioned his candidacy in passing. For example, one woman told me that another customer at Costco rammed her shopping cart into hers while she was speaking Spanish and told her to go back to her country. Others called Trump's incendiary rhetoric nonsense, but nobody seemed to think that he would be elected to lead the country in a few months' time. Once he was in office, a slew of anti-immigrant policies were quickly enacted, from those that restricted migration to the United States—or even travel, such as the Muslim ban—to the "public charge" rule by which seeking the most basic of services could have a negative impact on noncitizens' chances of obtaining a green card.[1]

Although the public charge policy would be substantially reduced in scope and eventually overturned in November 2020, it triggered memories of past policies, like Prop 187, that had sought to ban undocumented populations from accessing basic public services like health care and education in California. Multiple studies have detailed the chilling effects of the public charge rule on mixed-status and noncitizen families. One in four lower-income immigrant families in California stopped participating in or refrained from signing up for programs like food assistance and health care services for fear of the negative consequences for their bid for U.S. citizenship in the future.[2] Advocacy organizations had to scramble to push back against the public charge rule when it was leaked in a 2018 memo, and then they had to work to interpret the rule and educate the public on the resulting policies when it went into effect in February 2020.

Just one month later, the COVID-19 pandemic began. Stay-at-home orders were passed in California and eventually in the rest of the United States. Suddenly millions of people lost their jobs, were at risk of losing their homes, or had to contend with risking their health and their loved ones' health because they held essential jobs and were required to work. Latinx, Asian and Pacific Islander, Indigenous, and Black communities were among the hardest hit by the virus.[3]

During this time of crisis, millions of individuals and families felt the ramifications of a weak and limited safety net that was not built to buffer the population from the sudden fallout and economic downturn induced by the pandemic. People experienced delays of up to six months before they received unemployment benefits, and undocumented and mixed-status households were excluded from programs that could have helped cover their rent or pay for their next meal.[4] During this period of unprecedented need, some states, including California, slightly expanded their safety net programs, such as increasing monthly payments for food assistance through the Supplemental Nutrition Assistance Program (SNAP) and implementing two programs to aid undocumented individuals and families: Pandemic EBT (P-EBT, emergency food assistance for families with school-age children) and Disaster Relief Assistance for Immigrants (DRAI). Both programs were rolled out by the California Department of Social Services (CDSS) and funded in large part by foundation monies.[5] The amount allocated was a onetime payment of $500 per adult, with a maximum of $1,000 of aid per household, no matter its size. Although this payment was useful to the undocumented households in the states that implemented the program, they received less than one-sixth of what U.S. citizens and legal permanent residents received from the U.S. government in 2020: three payments of $1,200, $600, and $1,400 per individual (or $3,200 for a household of one) and $1,400 per child.

During the summer of 2020, as California began rolling out the emergency assistance, I consulted with a nonprofit organization that was tasked with implementing the P-EBT and DRAI programs. Over the course of four months, I had conversations over the phone with undocumented parents who had lost their jobs, who had lost their housing or feared losing their housing, and who were scrambling to find food for themselves and their children. I heard about a mother who was publicly shamed at a food bank and accused of lying when she said she had eight children. I heard from people who felt "cast aside" because they were not eligible for federal aid. I also saw firsthand how technological inequalities affected lower-income households that were expected to be online to learn about services, connect with them, and apply for different resources.[6]

The pandemic put into stark relief just how broken and conditional the U.S. safety net was and the disproportionate effects of its fissures on BIPOC communities. In California, it demonstrated that, during times of fiscal crisis, even a politically pro-immigrant state would deprioritize funding for programs directed at noncitizen and undocumented populations—such as when the state decided to not move forward with the expansion of Medi-Cal to undocumented individuals over the age of sixty-five in 2020.[7]

In 2021, the Biden administration ushered in new opportunities to strengthen and revitalize the safety net. The American Rescue Plan Act expanding the scope of existing safety net services during the COVID-19 pandemic was passed, an executive order to expand resources for advancing racial equity was issued, funding was approved for improving home energy costs at the state level, and the Bipartisan Infrastructure Law included $65 billion to make broadband internet more accessible.[8] All of these pandemic-related measures served to make the safety net more accessible. However, the Biden administration has pursued a mixed set of actions regarding immigration policy, sending unclear signals about the care that immigrants deserve to receive.[9]

Long-standing changes to the safety net will require a large cultural shift that fundamentally reimagines what the safety net provides, for whom, and to what end. This new framing would change the logic of exclusion and punishment into a logic of inclusion and care, thereby calling national borders, prisons, and racial hierarchies into question. As the stories of Tomás, Mari, Magdalena, Manuel, and many others in this book have shown, a more humane immigration and criminal justice system, complemented by a more inclusive safety net, would positively change millions of lives.

METHODOLOGICAL APPENDIX

I have heard from many scholars that the greatest challenge and reward in research is fieldwork, and I couldn't agree more. Undertaking a multi-sited project that sought to speak to the experiences of Spanish-speaking immigrants across at least three dimensions of difference (place, gender, and immigration status) proved to be more challenging but also more rewarding than I had anticipated. In this appendix, I provide a more detailed and humanized portrait of the research project in order to help and inform other students or scholars doing this work. Often missed in the methods of social science research is the day-to-day emotional labor and meaning-making that goes into it. I fill in some of the more intimate gaps in the research process here by giving a candid account of working "in the field," reflecting on how my positionality may have affected that process and being open about the strategies I used to handle emotionally tough moments and interviews. I end with some thoughts on how I would approach research projects differently in the future.

THE ASK: RECRUITING RESPONDENTS
FOR IN-DEPTH INTERVIEWS

The initial question that led to this research study was: How do social service providers respond to the increased demand for social services in the suburbs? To begin to answer it, I contacted nonprofit organizations that worked with immigrant populations in Oakland's eastern suburbs. I used resources like Guidestar to identify key immigrant organizations, and through interviews with staff members I learned more about other key organizations that worked with the Latinx immigrant community. Every person I spoke to was kind and enthusiastic about the study, a response that motivated me to give back in whatever way I could. I started volunteering as a bilingual intake interpreter for an NPO that provided food assistance by day, and I cotaught English and citizenship classes in the evenings. On weekends I went to citizenship workshops and attended Spanish mass at different churches. I enjoyed the ethnographic experience of these spaces, but I knew that eventually I would need to step forward and recruit people for interviews, which weren't going to conduct themselves.

After several weeks of observing and volunteering at an organization, I slowly but surely began asking NPO staff if I could recruit people for interviews for this study. Even though I was nervous each time I asked, many staff members were open to having me talk about this research, and they provided opportunities and spaces separate from my volunteer work where I could recruit people. For example, I was able to recruit many mothers with young children for interviews by coming into the center's after-parent meetings to talk about the study. Some centers provided me with a small room to conduct interviews inside the organization's building, making it easier for respondents to meet with me. Mothers talked to me while their children were tutored at the center. Day laborers talked to me while they waited for employers to come by worker centers. When I could not obtain a space at a center, I would offer to go to a respondent's home or to meet in a public space like a café or a park near where they worked or lived. The interviews in respondents' homes always proved to be the most fruitful, not only because we were in a safe, private space, but also because I could gain a better sense of their living situation and their family dynamics (although, admittedly, most of the home interviews were with women).

I was pleased that respondents trusted me and were willing to give their time and energy to an interview, but I worried that my recruitment method had led to a biased and selective sample. In an attempt to recruit a more extensive and potentially more varied sample for this research, I secured the permission of a prominent federally qualified health center to distribute flyers in Spanish to recruit people for interviews. Months after I had posted the flyers, however, not a single person had called expressing interest in participating in the study. I asked clinic staff if I could briefly introduce myself in clinic waiting rooms to present the study, but it was reasonably explained to me that this would be a disruption in services.

Given that recruiting people from posting flyers had been unsuccessful, I changed my recruiting method and tried to recruit respondents in person at different spaces. I spoke to street food vendors in Oakland about participating in the study, and I also frequented flea markets to recruit vendors for interviews. I scheduled meetings with priests to talk to them about the study and to ask for permission to make an announcement about the study during services. Every priest I spoke to was encouraging and interested in this research, and I was able to recruit respondents for interviews at three churches.

Once I had established relationships with several nonprofit organizations after one year of fieldwork, I participated in the Undergraduate Research Apprenticeship Program (URAP), which gave undergraduate students a chance to provide support to research projects in exchange for college credits. As part of this program, I trained undergraduates on how to conduct interviews, and they accompanied me as I conducted outreach to recruit participants at churches and flea markets. They served as notetakers for three interviews before having the opportunity to conduct interviews on their own. (Owing to students' and respondents' scheduling constraints, only one undergraduate student was able to conduct three interviews on her own.) I also provided training in creating interview guides, coding interviews, and analyzing interview data using qualitative research software, which we did as a group. I also cowrote an internal report for a day labor center with one of the undergraduate students who participated in URAP for an extra semester.

One of the contributions of this research design is the inclusion of people of varying immigration statuses to determine the influence of immigration status on their options and strategies for accessing services. I wanted a variety of experiences represented in this study, but I did not know how to ensure that. I certainly did not feel comfortable openly asking people for their immigration status, so I decided not to include questions on immigration status as part of the screening process for conducting interviews. Fortunately for me, people of all immigration statuses felt comfortable being interviewed by me, and surprisingly, I was also able to speak to a disproportionate number of people who had acquired, or were in the process of acquiring, a U-visa. Because they had already talked to a lawyer and sent in their application for the visa to U.S. Citizenship and Immigration Services, they felt assured that there was no harm done in talking to me because they had already disclosed their status to a U.S. legal entity. Interestingly enough, people with legal permanent resident status worried that their stories wouldn't be "helpful" to me, and they asked if I was sure I wanted to capture their story.

Sixteen respondents preferred not to have the interview recorded, but most of them felt comfortable with being recorded after I assured them that their identity would remain anonymous and I would delete the interviews from the audiotapes after transcribing them. I took several precautions to make sure that their story and personal information could not be traced back to them: I received verbal versus written consent for interviews; I asked only for their first names throughout the recruitment and interview process; in my field notes, I created and used pseudonyms for every individual I spoke with; I deleted each respondent's phone number from my phone after conducting the interview; and I stored all information in separate and password-protected files on an encrypted hard drive. That said, the fear of unintentionally putting respondents' privacy at risk stayed with me throughout the project—despite all the precautions and security measures I took.

POSITIONALITY

My position as a 1.5-generation Mexican immigrant and fluent native Spanish speaker made it easier for me to connect with respondents. We felt comfortable and familiar with each other during interviews, and the ease of communication may have made it possible for me to conduct these interviews in the first place. Many women would use the term of endearment *mija* with me, and some were eager to have me meet their daughters, so that I could talk to them about college. I did not meet too many respondents' children in the end, but when I did, I would ask them what year of school they were in or comment on an extracurricular activity their parent had mentioned, and I would ask them what colleges they were interested in (if their parent had mentioned that they were planning to go to college). I left my email address with them and said that I'd be happy to discuss any questions they had about college or school. I was not surprised, however, when no mentoring relationships developed from such brief interactions.

Women were the most likely to take me into their home for an interview, but they talked less about their immigration situation or their financial or emotional hardships than the men I interviewed. My guess is that men talked less often at length about themselves with others, and so this interview provided a space to process and reflect on their lives with an interested listener. Both men and women sometimes asked immigration questions that, feeling powerless, I was unable and unqualified to answer. I compiled a list of nearby nonprofit organizations that offered low-cost services, such as legal aid, medical care, childcare, classes, and food assistance, so that, at the very minimum, I could refer them to relevant NPOs. I included phone numbers on this list that they could call for referrals to different social services. That said, the information I supplied could go only so far; as this book has shown, personal connections and referrals were the most effective forms of outreach for services available to my respondents. Unlike many others in their networks, I had not used the services myself, so I was unable to share any personal experiences of seeking services at different organizations.

Many of the respondents were deeply religious, and as a self-identifying agnostic and culturally Catholic person, I felt a bit nervous at the thought of having my religiosity put to the test. With one minor exception, most respondents did not inquire into my own religious beliefs or faith; instead, they described the role that faith played in their lives. Some respondents would invite me into their congregation, and I would thank them for the invitation. That said, I did find myself praying more and becoming slightly more religious as I interacted with devout people of faith—a testament to the power of the social in shaping individual behavior.

An unexpected consequence of this fieldwork was being seen by some respondents as a financial resource for their businesses. Women in particular would give me their business card or show me jewelry that they sold to see if I would like to buy it. Normally this interaction would occur after the interview. I would politely look through their collection and ask them about how they started their business and how they ran it; this conversation gave me another opportunity to get to know them. I did not purchase any items from respondents, but I did provide financial compensation at the beginning of each interview, which was included in a handwritten card thanking them for their time.

Although I expected my white-presenting appearance to play a bigger role in how respondents opened up to or interacted with me, I found that most people did not question my Latinx identity once I spoke Spanish to them. Only one respondent thought I was ethnically white at the start of the interview, and she skeptically asked me why I was doing this project. When I told her that my own background as a Mexican immigrant had motivated me to do this research, she opened up and said that it made much more sense to her now.

Nevertheless, my light-skinned privilege, along with my class privilege and educational background, probably influenced my interactions with respondents in ways that were not perceptible to me. I am also not very knowledgeable about Indigenous history in Mexico and Central America, so when I spoke to respondents who were part of Indigenous groups and spoke an Indigenous language, like Ma'am or Mayan, it is likely that I missed much about the structures that had put them in a vulnerable position in their country of origin. This experience made me even more aware of the need for more Indigenous scholars and for a focus on Indigeneity in immigration research.[1]

RECOMMENDATIONS AND TAKEAWAYS
FOR FUTURE RESEARCH

Conducting my first large-scale research project was a continual learning experience. I had to push myself outside my comfort zone to recruit a diverse sample for interviews. Although it was useful to speak to respondents who were involved in nonprofit organizations, expanding my recruitment methods to encompass talking to street food vendors, flea market vendors, and priests, even if this style of recruitment made me nervous, brought me in contact with potential respondents who had a wider range of experiences.

In conducting interviews, I learned to be patient and accommodating with every person who was willing to devote time to talking to me. I came to understand that I could not take it personally if respondents missed or canceled an interview; when one respondent did so multiple times, I let the individual know that I would stop following up with them, but that the door was always open for them to reach out to me. Another best practice I discovered was to provide compensation for respondents' time at the beginning of an interview rather than at the end; that way, respondents did not feel pressured to finish an interview with me if they did not feel comfortable doing so.

I also had to recognize my limits as a researcher and prioritize self-care strategies while doing emotionally heavy fieldwork. After some interviews, I needed to go home and cry, or think, or just take a nap. I needed to allow myself to process everything. It was only after a period of processing and decompressing that I could find the clarity to identify and detail the essential components of an interview if it was recorded or to capture the whole of the interview by digitizing written notes if it was not recorded. To give myself this space to fully take in and respect each respondent's life experiences and narrative, I conducted just one or two interviews a day, with only a few exceptions.

Toward the end of this research project, I had the opportunity to collaborate with a nonprofit organization by writing an internal report on how its clients accessed different services, what organizational strategies worked well to facilitate access, and what strategies could use improvement. The findings from this internal report would later inform the NPO's grant proposals related to expanding its programs and funding. This more applied research proved to be one of the most rewarding parts of my experience. Going forward, I now know how to approach and ask organizations about the potential for such collaborations earlier in the research process. I also would like to incorporate into the research ways to share the findings with respondents, so that I could garner constructive feedback on what resonated with them and what did not, as well as hear their critiques or suggestions for future research.

I tried my best to capture the range of respondents' experiences honestly and fully, but as with any research project, my perspective cannot capture the full scope of the topic I examined. There is always room for more critique, interrogation, and growth.

The best research comes from a place of collective knowledge production, especially when it is led by those who are most impacted by the systems under examination. Although my arguments in this book offer a framework to think about the safety net, it is not the only possible framework, or the best framework, to understand the current fissures in the welfare state and their implications. Much of the knowledge about how the safety net operates in theory and in practice is currently being shared by those who have navigated it; many communities hold and shape this knowledge. I encourage all researchers and scholars to find ways to incorporate more participatory research approaches— or at a minimum, to build in feedback loops earlier in the research process— to ensure that they capture and share a full and nuanced picture of people's lived experiences. Better yet would be finding ways to enable people with those lived experiences to directly lead the work and tell their stories. The more power is ceded and shared in the research process, the more potential there is for individual and collective transformation in the validation, production, and sharing of knowledge to achieve change.

NOTES

INTRODUCTION

1. Minton and Giannarelli 2019.
2. Bohn et al. 2013; Herd and Moynihan 2019.
3. Fix 2009.
4. Chishti and Bolter 2020.
5. Budiman 2019; Hayes and Hill 2017.
6. Gee et al. 2017.
7. I use the term "Latinx" as a gender-inclusive alternative to Latino. While the gender-inclusive "Latine" fits more neatly with the Spanish language, the term "Latinx" has been in existence longer and has become more socialized in the United States as a gender-inclusive term (Vidal-Ortiz and Martínez, 2018).
8. Chavez 2013.
9. Fox 2019.
10. Dodd and Shelton 2021.
11. Nadasen 2007.
12. Minton and Giannarelli 2019.
13. Organization for Economic Cooperation and Development 2019.
14. Myles and Quadagno 2002.
15. Orloff and Skocpol 1984; Skocpol 1992. For more on the sociopolitical factors that shaped the origins of the U.S. welfare state, see Weir, Orloff, and Skocpol 1988 and Orloff 1993.
16. Skocpol 1992; Leff 1973.
17. Katznelson 2005.
18. Fox 2012.
19. Katznelson 2005.

20. Faber 2020.
21. Lei 2015. According to the Urban Institute (Lei 2015, updated with 2017 data), in 2016 the average wealth of White families, at $919,000, was seven times greater than the average wealth of Black families ($140,000) and five times greater than the average wealth of Latino families ($192,000). The racial wealth gap was not this large in 1963 (Schram et al. 2009).
22. Davis 1983.
23. Reese 2011.
24. Schram et al. 2009.
25. Curran and Abrams 2000.
26. Hamer and Marchioro 2002.
27. Geva 2011.
28. Dill, Zinn, and Patton 1999.
29. Barnett 2018.
30. Fox 2019.
31. Nadasen 2007.
32. Henderson and Tickamyer 2009.
33. Brown 2015; Hohle 2017; Newfield 2011.
34. Stack 1974; Edin and Lein 1997.
35. Soss 2000b.
36. Jones-Correa 1998.
37. Coll 2010; Gast and Okamoto 2016; Yoshikawa 2011.
38. Most of the Antioch interviews were conducted with residents of that suburb, but I also spoke to four respondents from the neighboring suburbs of Pittsburg, Martinez, and Bay Point.
39. Moskowitz 2017.
40. Allard and Paisner 2016.
41. For more on how race and immigration status intersect, see Cacho 2012; Cho 2017; Loyd and Mountz 2018; Ngai 2014.
42. One respondent was raised in Nicaragua and one in Honduras, but most Central American respondents came from Guatemala and El Salvador.
43. For more on Indigenous history in the United States, California, and the Bay Area up to the present day, see Dunbar-Ortiz 2014; Keliiaa 2021; Lindsay 2012.
44. Henderson 2011.
45. Ibid.
46. Ibid.

47. Ibid.
48. Johnson 2001.
49. O'Connor, Batalova, and Bolter 2019.
50. Leogrande 1990.
51. Individuals with a green card have been granted long-term residency status and are allowed to seek formal employment in the United States. After five years, they may apply for U.S. citizenship. Those who are granted asylum status are allowed to stay in the United States as long as the U.S. government still deems their country of origin too dangerous to return to. After one year of asylum status, individuals can apply for a green card (legal permanent residency status). U-visas, designed for victims of domestic crime, initially allow the holder to access some public benefits, to work legally in the United States, and to apply, after three years, for legal permanent residency status. This visa status contrasts with TPS, which does not allow for a path toward permanent residency or citizenship. TPS must be renewed (for a costly fee) every year. Moreover, it can be terminated at any point, rendering former TPS holders undocumented.
52. Médecins Sans Frontiers 2017.
53. Vogt 2018.
54. U.S. Citizenship and Immigration Services 2022.
55. Garip 2012. For more on current patterns and motivations for migration, see Asad and Garip 2019.
56. Menjívar 2000.
57. I detail percentages here and in other sections of the book merely to show how often patterns showed up in the data; they are not statistically representative of the population on which this study focuses.
58. Babey et al. 2021.

CHAPTER 1
CONDITIONAL CARE: THE EXCLUSION OF VULNERABLE POPULATIONS FROM PUBLIC BENEFITS

1. Goldman, Smith, and Sood 2005.
2. Calvo, Jablonska-Bayro, and Waters 2017.
3. Cooper 2015.
4. Alexander 2011, 16.
5. Clabaugh 2004.

6. Fox 2019.
7. Nadeem et al. 2007; Wroe 2008.
8. Kornbluh and Mink 2019; Schram et al. 2009. The PRWORA restrictions apply only to legal permanent residents who arrived in the United States after August 22, 1996. Legal permanent residents who arrived before that date are still eligible for public programs.
9. Fix and Passel 2002.
10. Lichter and Crowley 2004.
11. Kaushal and Kaestner 2005; Van Hook and Balistreri 2006.
12. Altman, Stephens, and Yates 2012.
13. Centers for Medicare and Medicaid Services 2022; Kaiser Family Foundation 2023.
14. Cha and McConville 2021.
15. Broder 2023.
16. U.S. Census Bureau, n.d.-e, n.d.-f, n.d.-g.
17. For MIT's calculations, see the "Living Wage Calculator" at https://livingwage .mit.edu.
18. Berlinger and Gusmano 2013.
19. Broder 2023.
20. Molina 2011; Park 2011.
21. Wakefield 2021.
22. Human Resources and Safety Administration, "Health Center Program: Impact and Growth," updated August 2022, https://bphc.hrsa.gov/about/healthcenter program.
23. Centers for Medicare and Medicaid Services, "Federally Qualified Health Centers (FHQC) Center," https://www.cms.gov/Center/Provider-Type/Federally-Qualified -Health-Centers-FQHC-Center.
24. Alameda County, CA 2014.
25. Applied Survey Research 2022.
26. California Primary Care Association 2017.
27. California Pan-Ethnic Health Network 2019, 15; California Primary Care Association 2017.
28. California Pan-Ethnic Health Network 2019.
29. Slack and Martínez 2018.
30. Kulish 2018.
31. Rasmussen et al. 2007.
32. Rank 2010.
33. Gehi 2012.

34. Perreira and Ornelas 2013.

35. Koech et al. 2022.

36. Schanzenbach and Tomeh 2020.

37. Myers and Painter 2017; Walsemann, Ro, and Gee 2017.

38. Castañeda and Melo 2014.

39. Castner, Mabli, and Sykes 2009.

40. U.S. Department of Agriculture 2019.

41. Long 2002.

42. Neuberger and Greenstein 2004.

43. Chauvenet et al. 2019.

44. Fine 2006; *Philadelphia Inquirer* 2021.

45. Monforton and Von Bergen 2021.

46. Griffith 2015.

CHAPTER 2
PLACE-BASED ACCESS TO CARE

1. Kneebone and Berube 2014a.

2. Singer, Hardwick, and Bretell 2008.

3. Allard 2008; Murphy 2010; Murphy and Wallace 2010; Weir et al. 2012.

4. De Graauw, Gleeson, and Bloemraad 2013; Joassart-Marcelli 2013; Panchok-Berry, Rivas, and Murphy 2013; Roth and Allard 2016.

5. Moskowitz 2017.

6. Schafran 2019.

7. Ibid.

8. Opillard 2015.

9. U.S. Census Bureau, n.d.-d.

10. Kneebone and Berube 2014b; KQED 2017; Palomino 2015 (updated 2016).

11. U.S. Census Bureau 2020f, n.d.-c.

12. Data USA, Oakland, California profile, data taken from U.S. Census Bureau 2020, https://datausa.io/profile/geo/oakland-ca (accessed September 2023).

13. As a practitioner and staff member of a Non-Profit Organization, NPO is the term most used in my field in contrast to NGO or Non-Governmental-Organization.

14. Candid, "Guidestar," https://www.guidestar.org/ (accessed July 16, 2022).

15. The Health Program of Alameda County (HealthPAC) is a countywide program that offers basic health services for residents of Alameda who are at or below the 200 percent FPL, are not enrolled in full-scope Medi-Cal, and do not have insurance through a private provider. The services offered through this program

include wellness checkups and preventative services, illness and injury care, care for ongoing health issues, mental health care and health education, and prescriptions for medicine. Copays for services are based on income. For more information, see HealthPAC 2018.

16. U.S. Census Bureau 2020e.

17. U.S. Census. n.d.-b.

18. Ibid.

19. See California Housing Partnership and Urban Displacement Project 2018 for a more detailed understanding of the housing infrastructure in Contra Costa County. See Schafran 2019 for a more detailed overview of the political landscape that shapes current housing and zoning laws in the Bay Area.

20. U.S. Census Bureau 2020d.

21. Candid, "Guidestar," https://www.guidestar.org/ (accessed July 16, 2022).

22. California Department of Health Care Access and Information (HCAI), "FQHC List Public," https://funding.hcai.ca.gov/fqhc-site-search/ (accessed May 27, 2022).

23. An accredited BIA representative is a non-attorney who has the capacity to represent clients before the BIA, the U.S. Department of Homeland Security (DHS), or both.

24. Pedro's mention of grant funding reflects the larger trend of public interest law firms increasingly being funded by governmental grants, which can restrict the types of services they are able to provide and to whom (Albiston and Nielsen 2014).

25. U.S. Census Bureau, n.d.-a, n.d.-b., n.d.-c.

26. Since the study was conducted, the resources for low-cost immigration legal aid remain the same. The organizational websites indicate that at least fifty-three staff members work at NPOs in Oakland (including attorneys, interpreters, interns, paralegals, and legal and administrative assistants), compared to only five known staff members so employed near Antioch (and only one is a staff attorney). Also since the study, the satellite legal aid office in Antioch moved to an office in the more rural nearby town of Brentwood.

27. Cervantes and Menjívar 2020.

28. Lowrey 2021.

29. Stutzer and Frey 2008.

30. Vidal de Haymes, O'Donoghue, and Nguyen 2019.

31. This kind of response to a victim of crime was described one time in interviews, so I cannot determine the motives for these police officers' behavior in this one incident, nor how representative it was of the whole Walnut Creek police department.

32. Castleman 2023.

33. De Graauw and Gleeson 2021.

CHAPTER 3
"SHE WAS THE ONE THAT MOVED ME": NETWORKS
AND PARENTHOOD AS CONDITIONS FOR CARE

1. Soss 2000b.
2. Abel 2004.
3. Mayorkas 2021.
4. National Immigration Law Center 2017.
5. Hennessy-Fiske 2015.
6. Molina 2011.
7. Carcamo 2013.
8. Marrow 2009.
9. Living in a mixed-status household, such as Asunción's, elicits different power dynamics and complications for immigrant families; these issues are explored in more detail in, for example, Dreby 2019 and Menjívar, Abrego, and Schmalzbauer 2016.
10. Calvo, Jablonska-Bayro, and Waters 2017.
11. Massey 1999.
12. Menjívar 2000.
13. Zhou 2009.
14. De Souza Briggs, Popkin, and Goering 2010.
15. Ibid.
16. On NPOs and individuals' social capital, see Small 2009. On NPOs as catalysts for collective mobilization, see Bloemraad and Terriquez 2016; Coll 2010.
17. Soss 2000b.
18. Coll 2010.
19. Desmond and Travis 2018.
20. On restrictions related to residency, see Beckett and Herbert 2009; Goffman 2009. On restricted public benefits, see Harding et al. 2014.
21. Jones-Correa 1998.

CHAPTER 4
"I DON'T HAVE ANYTHING. NO DOCTOR . . . NO NOTHING":
LABOR AND CRISES AS CONDITIONS FOR CARE

1. Berg and Upchurch 2007; Rook et al. 2011.
2. Galdas, Cheater, and Marshall 2005.

3. Courtenay 2000.
4. Lohan 2007.
5. For comparisons of Latino and Black men to White men, see Cheatham, Barksdale, and Rodgers 2008; for comparisons to Latina and Black women, see Williams 2003.
6. Cabassa 2007.
7. Cha and McConville 2021.
8. Kaiser Family Foundation 2023.
9. Ro, Van Hook, and Walsemann 2022.
10. Hadley 2003.
11. Kaiser Family Foundation 2023.
12. Holmes 2013.
13. Hansen and Donohoe 2003; Villarejo and McCurdy 2008.
14. Holmes 2013.
15. Valenzuela et al. 2006, 3.
16. Molina 2006.
17. Park 2011.
18. Black 2003.
19. Stern 2005.
20. Ibid.
21. Molina 2006.
22. Mujeres Unidas y Activas, Day Labor Program Women's Collective of La Raza Centro Legal, and DataCenter 2007.
23. Asad and Clair 2016.
24. Holmes 2013.
25. Gleeson 2010.
26. This interview took place before the COVID-19 pandemic, a time when the decision to go to work despite cold symptoms seemed less complicated to many people.
27. At the onset of the 2009 recession, primary care services were cut in California for undocumented adults. Although primary care services were restored in 2015 through the Contra Costa Cares program, this program is more limited in scope and funding. Only three thousand participants are allowed, and they are enrolled on a first-come, first-served basis through screenings at four medical sites in the county. None of the men I interviewed knew about Contra Costa Cares, and only one woman residing in Contra Costa County participated in it, after being referred by a nonprofit.

28. Even though the state of California has passed laws to prevent collusion between ICE and law enforcement agencies, these agencies continue to collude by exploiting loopholes in these laws. Stricter laws have been put forward to close these loopholes (Romani 2022).

CHAPTER 5
"WE GIVE THE BEST TO THE COUNTRY, BUT THE COUNTRY IS NOT READY TO GIVE THE BEST TO US": ENGAGING THE LOGIC OF CONDITIONAL CARE

1. Abrego 2011.
2. Internal Revenue Service, "About Earned Income Tax Credit & Other Refundable Credits," https://www.eitc.irs.gov/eitc-central/about-eitc/about-eitc (accessed July 25, 2020).
3. Ross 2016. In announcing in 2015 that he was running for president, Donald Trump said that Mexican immigrants brought drugs and crime into the United States and were rapists. He used similar language in the third and final presidential debate when he vowed to secure the borders and get rid of "bad hombres."
4. Wimmer 2008.
5. For more on the experiences of transnational families, see Abrego 2014.
6. Anti-Blackness attitudes and colorism are prominent throughout much of Central and Latin America, including Mexico, which could influence the boundary-making narratives we see here. For more on the history of anti-Blackness and colorism in Latin America and guidelines to combat it, see Adames, Chavez-Dueñas, and Jernigan 2021.
7. Andrews 2017.
8. O'Toole 2020. Deferred Action for Childhood Arrivals, passed in 2012, is only a temporary order; it offers no pathway to citizenship and may not safeguard against deportation. The temporary and fleeting nature of DACA was cast into high relief when it was rescinded in September 2017. It was upheld by the U.S. Supreme Court in June 2020, but as of July 6, 2022, U.S. Citizenship and Immigration Services (USCIS) was still not processing new applications.
9. Scott 1990.
10. Scott 1985.
11. Lamont 2000.
12. Fleming, Lamont, and Welburn 2012.
13. Asad and Clair 2018; Williams, Lawrence, and Davis 2019.
14. Seif 2014.
15. Gallo 2016; Muñoz and Maldonado 2012.

16. Coll 2010.
17. Gleeson 2010.
18. Asad 2020a.
19. Bloemraad, Voss, and Silva 2014.
20. Haynes, Merolla, and Ramakrishnan 2016.

CHAPTER 6
CONCLUSION: MOVING TOWARD
UNCONDITIONAL CARE

1. Soss 2002a; Soss, Fording, and Schram 2011.
2. Edin and Lein 1997.
3. Coll 2010; Yoshikawa 2011.
4. Asad and Garip 2019; Garip 2012.
5. Allard 2017; De Graauw, Gleeson, and Bloemraad 2013; Joassart-Marcelli 2013; Murphy and Wallace 2010; Panchok-Berry, Rivas, and Murphy 2013.
6. García Hernández 2014; Stumpf 2006.
7. Alvord, Menjívar, and Cervantes 2018; Andrews 2018; Asad and Rosen 2018; Babey et al. 2021; Capps et al. 2007; García 2020; Prieto 2018.
8. Alvord, Menjívar, and Cervantes 2018; Andrews 2018; Asad and Rosen 2018; Prieto 2018; Asad 2020b.
9. As of the time of this writing, federal policy advises against enforcing immigration-related laws in "sensitive areas," such as health centers, courts, schools, and churches.
10. Chishti and Bolter 2017.
11. Fix 2009; Fox 2016.
12. Acosta et al. 2020; Baker and Marchevsky 2019; Fleming et al. 2017; Golash-Boza and Hondagneu-Sotelo 2013.
13. Moynihan, Herd, and Harvey 2014.
14. Rosales 2020.
15. Menjívar 2000.
16. Cervantes and Menjívar 2020.
17. Cho 2017.
18. Louie, Kim, and Chan 2020.
19. Cho 2017.
20. Alvord, Menjívar, and Cervantes 2018; Andrews 2018; Asad and Rosen 2018; De Graauw and Gleeson 2016; Prieto 2018.
21. Golash-Boza and Hondagneu-Sotelo 2013.
22. Cervantes and Menjívar 2020; García and Schmalzbauer 2017; Schmalzbauer 2014.

23. For more on the intersection of Indigeneity and migration, see Asad and Hwang 2018. For more on differences between Mexican and Central American migrants, see Menjívar and Abrego 2012. For more on LGBTQIA+ populations, see Seif 2016.
24. Immigrant Legal Resource Center 2022.
25. Office of Governor Gavin Newsom 2022.
26. Sosa 2022.
27. For more on county-level health programs for immigrants in California, see Health Access 2015.
28. Allard 2019.
29. De Graauw 2016.
30. Monforton and Von Bergen 2021.
31. Délano Alonso 2018; Osorio, Dávila, and Castañeda 2019.
32. Mission Asset Fund, "Financial Equity Framework: A Solution Rooted in Community," https://www.missionassetfund.org/financial-equity-framework/.
33. Esping-Andersen 2002; Finch 2021; Saxonberg 2013.
34. Nicholls, Maussen, and Caldas de Mesquita 2016.
35. Haynes, Merolla, and Ramakrishnan 2016.
36. Molina 2006, 2011.
37. University of California–Los Angeles 2022.
38. Bernhardt et al. 2008; Doussard 2013; Weil 2014.
39. On UBI experiments, see Hasdell 2020. On restitutive housing program experiments, see Fairbanks 2022.

EPILOGUE
1. Chishti and Bolter 2017.
2. Babey et al. 2021.
3. Webb Hooper, Nápoles, and Pérez-Stable 2020.
4. Finney and Koury 2021.
5. Suro and Findling 2020.
6. Cherewka 2020.
7. Torres-Pinzon et al. 2020. The following year, the Office of the Governor expanded Medi-Cal access to eligible adults age fifty and older, regardless of immigration status, and it took effect in May 2022.
8. U.S. Department of the Treasury 2021; Vollinger 2022; White House 2021, 2022.
9. Chishti and Bolter 2022.

METHODOLOGICAL APPENDIX
1. For more on migration and Indigeneity, see Asad and Hwang 2018.

REFERENCES

Abel, Emily K. 2004. "'Only the Best Class of Immigration': Public Health Policy toward Mexicans and Filipinos in Los Angeles, 1910–1940." *American Journal of Public Health* 94(6, June): 932–39. DOI: https://doi.org/10.2105/ajph.94.6.932.

Abrego, Leisy J. 2011. "Legal Consciousness of Undocumented Latinos: Fear and Stigma as Barriers to Claims-Making for First- and 1.5-Generation Immigrants." *Law and Society Review* 45(2, June): 337–70. DOI: https://doi.org/10.1111/j.1540-5893.2011.00435.x.

———. 2014. *Sacrificing Families: Navigating Laws, Labor, and Love across Borders.* Redwood City, Calif.: Stanford University Press.

Acosta, Laura M., Arthur R. Andrews, M. Natalia Acosta Canchila, and Athena K. Ramos. 2020. "Testing Traditional Machismo and the Gender Role Strain Theory with Mexican Migrant Farmworkers." *Hispanic Journal of Behavioral Sciences* 42(2, May): 215–34. DOI: https://doi.org/10.1177/0739986320915649.

Adames, Hector Y., Nayeli Y. Chavez-Dueñas, and Maryam M. Jernigan. 2021. "The Fallacy of a Raceless Latinidad: Action Guidelines for Centering Blackness in Latinx Psychology." *Journal of Latinx Psychology* 9(1, February): 26–44. DOI: https://doi.org/10.1037/lat0000179.

Alameda County, CA. 2014. "Community Screening and Enrolling Sites for the Uninsured." Updated July 17, 2014. http://achealthcare.org/health-insurance-info/low-income-coverage-options/screeningenrollment/ (accessed December 4, 2021).

Albiston, Catherine R., and Laura Beth Nielsen. 2014. "Funding the Cause: How Public Interest Law Organizations Fund Their Activities and Why It Matters for Social Change." *Law and Social Inquiry* 39(1, Winter): 62–95. DOI: https://doi.org/10.1111/lsi.12013.

Alexander, Michelle. 2011. "The New Jim Crow." *Ohio State Journal of Criminal Law* 9(1): 7–26.

Allard, Scott W. 2008. *Out of Reach: Place, Poverty, and the New American Welfare State.* New Haven, Conn.: Yale University Press.

———. 2017. *Places in Need: The Changing Geography of Poverty.* New York: Russell Sage Foundation.

———. 2019. "Spatial Patterns of Work, Poverty, and Safety Net Provision in the U.S." Final report presented to the US2050 Initiative, March 4. https://www .pgpf.org/sites/default/files/US-2050-Spatial-Patterns-of-Work-Poverty-and-Safety -Net-Provision-in-the-US.pdf.

Allard, Scott W., and Sarah Charnes Paisner. 2016. "The Rise of Suburban Poverty." *Oxford Handbook Topics in Politics* (September 1). DOI: https://doi.org/10.1093 /oxfordhb/9780199935307.013.96.

Altman, Stephanie, Gene Stephens, and Annika Yates. 2012. "The Invisible Uninsured: Non-Citizens and Access to Health Care Coverage under the Affordable Care Act." *Public Interest Law Reporter* 17(Summer): 230. http://lawecommons.luc.edu/pilr /vol17/iss3/6.

Alvord, Daniel R., Cecilia Menjívar, and Andrea Gómez Cervantes. 2018. "The Legal Violence in the 2017 Executive Orders: The Expansion of Immigrant Criminal-ization in Kansas." *Social Currents* 5(5, October): 411–20. DOI: https://doi.org /10.1177/2329496518762001.

Andrews, Abigail L. 2017. "Moralizing Regulation: The Implications of Policing 'Good' versus 'Bad' Immigrants." *Ethnic and Racial Studies* 41(14): 1–19. DOI: https://doi.org/10.1080/01419870.2017.1375133.

———. 2018. *Undocumented Politics: Place, Gender, and the Pathways of Mexican Migrants.* Berkeley: University of California Press.

Applied Survey Research. 2022. "2022 Alameda County: Homeless Count and Survey Comprehensive Report." https://everyonehome.org/wp-content/uploads/2022/12 /2022-Alameda-County-PIT-Report_9.22.22-FINAL-3.pdf.

Asad, Asad L. 2020a. "On the Radar: System Embeddedness and Latin American Immigrants' Perceived Risk of Deportation." *Law and Society Review* 54(1, March): 133–67. DOI: https://doi.org/10.1111/lasr.12460.

———. 2020b. "Latinos' Deportation Fears by Citizenship and Legal Status, 2007 to 2018." *Proceedings of the National Academy of Sciences of the United States of America* 117(16, April 21): 8836–44. DOI: https://doi.org/10.1073/pnas.1915460117.

Asad, Asad L., and Matthew Clair. 2018. "Racialized Legal Status as a Social Deter-minant of Health." *Social Science and Medicine* 199(February): 19–28. DOI: https://doi.org/10.1016/j.socscimed.2017.03.010.

Asad, Asad L., and Filiz Garip. 2019. "Mexico-U.S. Migration in Time: From Economic to Social Mechanisms." *Annals of the American Academy of Political and Social Science* 684(1, July): 60–84. DOI: https://doi.org/10.1177/0002716219847148.

Asad, Asad L., and Jackelyn Hwang. 2018. "Indigenous Places and the Making of Undocumented Status in Mexico-U.S. Migration." *International Migration Review* 53(4, December): 1032–77. DOI: https://doi.org/10.1177/0197918318801059.

Asad, Asad L., and Eva Rosen. 2018. "Hiding within Racial Hierarchies: How Undocumented Immigrants Make Residential Decisions in an American City." *Journal of Ethnic and Migration Studies* 45(11): 1857–82. DOI: https://doi.org/10.1080/1369183X.2018.1532787.

Babey, Susan, Joelle Wolstein, Riti Shimkhada, and Ninez Ponce. 2021. "One in 4 Low-Income Immigrant Adults in California Avoided Public Programs, Likely Worsening Food Insecurity and Access to Health Care." *Health Policy Brief.* UCLA Center for Health Policy Research, March. https://healthpolicy.ucla.edu/publications/Documents/PDF/2021/publiccharge-policybrief-mar2021.pdf.

Baker, Beth, and Alejandra Marchevsky. 2019. "Gendering Deportation, Policy Violence, and Latino/a Family Precarity." *Latino Studies* 17(2, June 1): 207–24. DOI: https://doi.org/10.1057/s41276-019-00176-0.

Barnett, Matt J. 2018. "Queering the Welfare State: Paradigmatic Heteronormativity after Obergefell." *New York University Law Review* 93(6, December): 1633–67.

Bay Area Census. n.d.-a. "City of Antioch Decennial Census Data: 1970–2010." http://www.bayareacensus.ca.gov/cities/Antioch.htm (accessed September 2023).

———. n.d.-b. "City of Concord Decennial Census Data: 1970–2010." http://www.bayareacensus.ca.gov/cities/Concord.htm (accessed September 2023).

———. n.d.-c. "City of Oakland Decennial Census Data: 1970–2010." http://www.bayareacensus.ca.gov/cities/Oakland.htm (accessed September 2023).

Beckett, Katherine, and Steve Herbert. 2009. *Banished: The New Social Control in America.* Oxford: Oxford University Press.

Berg, Cynthia A., and Renn Upchurch. 2007. "A Developmental-Contextual Model of Couples Coping with Chronic Illness across the Adult Life Span." *Psychological Bulletin* 133(6, November): 920–54. DOI: https://doi.org/10.1037/0033-2909.133.6.920.

Berlinger, Nancy, and Michael K. Gusmano. 2013. "Undocumented Patients: Undocumented Immigrants and Access to Health Care." Executive Summary. Hastings Center, March.

Bernhardt, Annette D., Heather Boushey, Laura Dresser, and Chris Tilly, eds. 2008. *The Gloves-Off Economy: Workplace Standards at the Bottom of America's Labor Market.* Ithaca, N.Y.: Cornell University Press.

Black, Edwin. 2003. *War against the Weak: Eugenics and America's Campaign to Create a Master Race*. Washington, D.C.: Dialog Press.

Bloemraad, Irene, and Veronica Terriquez. 2016. "Cultures of Engagement: The Organizational Foundations of Advancing Health in Immigrant and Low-Income Communities of Color." *Social Science and Medicine* 165(September): 214–22. DOI: https://doi.org/10.1016/j.socscimed.2016.02.003.

Bloemraad, Irene, Kim Voss, and Fabiana Silva. 2014. "Framing the Immigrant Movement as about Rights, Family, or Economics: Which Appeals Resonate and for Whom?" Institute for Research on Labor and Employment, May 1. https://escholarship.org/uc/item/3b32w33p.

Bohn, Sarah, Caroline Danielson, Matt Levin, Marybeth Mattingly, and Christopher Wimer. 2013. "The California Poverty Measure: A New Look at the Social Safety Net." Public Policy Institute of California, October. https://www.ppic.org/wp-content/uploads/content/pubs/report/R_1013SBR.pdf.

Broder, Tanya. 2023. "Table: Medical Assistance Programs for Immigrants in Various States." National Immigration Law Center, July 2021; updated March 2023. https://www.nilc.org/issues/health-care/medical-assistance-various-states/.

Brown, Wendy. 2015. *Undoing the Demos: Neoliberalism's Stealth Revolution*. New York: Zone Books.

Budiman, Abby. 2019. "Key Findings about U.S. Immigrants." Pew Research Center, August 20. https://www.pewresearch.org/?p=290738.

Cabassa, Leopoldo J. 2007. "Latino Immigrant Men's Perceptions of Depression and Attitudes toward Help Seeking." *Hispanic Journal of Behavioral Sciences* 29(4, November): 492–509. DOI: https://doi.org/10.1177/0739986307307157.

Cacho, Lisa Marie. 2012. *Social Death: Racialized Rightlessness and the Criminalization of the Unprotected*. New York: New York University Press.

California Housing Partnership and Urban Displacement Project. 2018. "Rising Housing Costs and Re-Segregation in Contra Costa County." https://chpc.wpenginepowered.com/wp-content/uploads/2018/09/CCResegregationReport_2018.pdf.

California Pan-Ethnic Health Network. 2019. "Accessing Mental Health in the Shadows: How Immigrants in California Struggle to Get Needed Care." February 2. https://cpehn.org/assets/uploads/archive/resource_files/cpehn_immigrant_mental_health_final3.pdf.

California Primary Care Association. 2017. "Leveraging Federally Qualified Health Centers in California's Behavioral Health Care Continuum." November 6. https://hcpsocal.org/wp-content/uploads/2018/05/Leveraging-FQHCs-in-CA-BH-Care-Continuum.pdf.

Calvo, Rocío, Joanna M. Jablonska-Bayro, and Mary C. Waters. 2017. "Obamacare in Action: How Access to the Health Care System Contributes to Immigrants' Sense of Belonging." *Journal of Ethnic and Migration Studies* 43(12): 1–17. DOI: https://doi.org/10.1080/1369183X.2017.1323449.

Capps, Randy, Rosa Maria Castañeda, Ajay Chaudry, and Robert Santos. 2007. *Paying the Price: The Impact of Immigration Raids on America's Children.* Urban Institute and National Council de la Raza, October 31. https://www.urban.org/sites/default/files/publication/46811/411566-Paying-the-Price-The-Impact-of-Immigration-Raids-on-America-s-Children.PDF.

Carcamo, Cindy. 2013. "Arizona Bill Would Compel Hospitals to Check Immigration Status." *Los Angeles Times*, January 26. http://articles.latimes.com/2013/jan/26/nation/la-na-nn-ff-arizona-hospitals-immigrants-20130125 (accessed January 5, 2016).

Carrillo, Dani. 2018. "Navigating Aid: Latinx Immigrants Accessing Services in a Post Welfare Reform Era." Ph.D. diss., University of California, Berkeley.

Castañeda, Heide, and Milena Andrea Melo. 2014. "Health Care Access for Latino Mixed-Status Families: Barriers, Strategies, and Implications for Reform." *American Behavioral Scientist* 58(14, December): 1891–1909. DOI: https://doi.org/10.1177/0002764214550290.

Castleman, Terry. 2023. "Antioch Police Department Mired in Racism Allegations—First in Text Messages, Now in a Brutality Lawsuit." *Los Angeles Times*, April 27.

Castner, Laura, James Mabli, and Julie Sykes. 2009. "Dynamics of WIC Program Participation by Infants and Children, 2001 to 2003. Final Report." Mathematica Policy Research. https://naldc.nal.usda.gov/catalog/43338.

Centers for Medicare and Medicaid Services (CMS). 2022. "March 2022 Medicaid and CHIP Enrollment Trends Snapshot." https://www.medicaid.gov/medicaid/national-medicaid-chip-program-information/downloads/march-2022-medicaid-chip-enrollment-trend-snapshot.pdf.

Cervantes, Andrea Gómez, and Cecilia Menjívar. 2020. "Legal Violence, Health, and Access to Care: Latina Immigrants in Rural and Urban Kansas." *Journal of Health and Social Behavior* 61(3, September): 307–23. DOI: https://doi.org/10.1177/0022146520945048.

Cha, Paulette, and Shannon McConville. 2021. "Health Coverage and Care for Undocumented Immigrants: An Update." Public Policy Institute of California, June. https://www.ppic.org/wp-content/uploads/health-coverage-and-care-for-undocumented-immigrants-in-california-june-2021.pdf.

Chauvenet, Christina, Molly De Marco, Carolyn Barnes, and Alice S. Ammerman. 2019. "WIC Recipients in the Retail Environment: A Qualitative Study Assessing

Customer Experience and Satisfaction." *Journal of the Academy of Nutrition and Dietetics* 119(3, March): 416–24. DOI: https://doi.org/10.1016/j.jand .2018.09.003.

Chavez, Leo. 2013. *The Latino Threat: Constructing Immigrants, Citizens, and the Nation.* Palo Alto, Calif.: Stanford University Press.

Cheatham, Cessaly T., Debra J. Barksdale, and Shielda G. Rodgers. 2008. "Barriers to Health Care and Health-Seeking Behaviors Faced by Black Men." *Journal of the American Academy of Nurse Practitioners* 20(11, November): 555–62. DOI: https://doi.org/10.1111/j.1745-7599.2008.00359.x.

Cherewka, Alexis. 2020. "The Digital Divide Hits U.S. Immigrant Households Disproportionately during the COVID-19 Pandemic." Migration Policy Institute, September 3. https://www.immigrationresearch.org/system/files/The%20Digital%20 Divide%20Hits%20U.S.%20Immigrant%20Households%20Disproportionately %20during%20the%20COVID-19%20Pandemic_0_0.pdf.

Chishti, Muzaffar, and Jessica Bolter. 2017. "The Trump Administration at Six Months: A Sea Change in Immigration Enforcement." Migration Policy Institute, July 19. https://www.migrationpolicy.org/article/trump-administration-six-months-sea -change-immigration-enforcement.

———. 2020. "Vulnerable to COVID-19 and in Frontline Jobs, Immigrants Are Mostly Shut Out of U.S. Relief." Migration Policy Institute, April 24. https:// www.migrationpolicy.org/article/covid19-immigrants-shut-out-federal-relief.

———. 2022. "Biden at the One-Year Mark: A Greater Change in Direction on Immigration Than Is Recognized." Migration Policy Institute, January 19. https:// www.migrationpolicy.org/article/biden-one-year-mark.

Cho, Esther Yoona. 2017. "Revisiting Ethnic Niches: A Comparative Analysis of the Labor Market Experiences of Asian and Latino Undocumented Young Adults." *RSF: The Russell Sage Foundation Journal of the Social Sciences* 3(4): 97–115. DOI: https://doi.org/10.7758/rsf.2017.3.4.06.

Clabaugh, Gary K. 2004. "The Educational Legacy of Ronald Reagan." *Educational Horizons* 82(4): 256–59.

Coll, Kathleen. 2010. *Remaking Citizenship: Latina Immigrants and New American Politics.* Palo Alto, Calif.: Stanford University Press.

Cooper, Hannah L. F. 2015. "War on Drugs Policing and Police Brutality." *Substance Use and Misuse* 50(8/9): 1188–94. DOI: https://doi.org/10.3109/10826084.2015 .1007669.

Courtenay, Will H. 2000. "Constructions of Masculinity and Their Influence on Men's Well-being: A Theory of Gender and Health." *Social Science and Medicine* 50(10, May): 1385–1401. DOI: https://doi.org/10.1016/s0277-9536(99)00390-1.

Curran, Laura, and Laura S. Abrams. 2000. "Making Men into Dads." *Gender & Society* 14(5): 662–78. DOI: https://doi.org/10.1177/089124300014005005.

Davis, Angela. 1983. *Women, Race, and Class.* New York: Vintage Press.

De Graauw, Els. 2016. *Making Immigrant Rights Real: Nonprofits and the Politics of Integration in San Francisco.* Ithaca, N.Y.: Cornell University Press.

De Graauw, Els, and Shannon Gleeson. 2016. "An Institutional Examination of the Local Implementation of the DACA Program." Working paper. Baruch College School of Public Affairs, Center for Nonprofit Strategy and Management, April. https://marxe.baruch.cuny.edu/wp-content/uploads/sites/7/2020/04/DeGraauwGleeson_ExaminationoflocalimplementationofDACA.pdf.

———. 2021. "Metropolitan Context and Immigrant Rights Experiences: DACA Awareness and Support in Houston." *Urban Geography* 42(8): 1119–46. DOI: https://doi.org/10.1080/02723638.2020.1752988.

De Graauw, Els, Shannon Gleeson, and Irene Bloemraad. 2013. "Funding Immigrant Organizations: Suburban Free Riding and Local Civic Presence." *American Journal of Sociology* 119(1, July): 75–130. https://www.journals.uchicago.edu/doi/epdf/10.1086/671168.

Délano Alonso, Alexandra. 2018. *From Here and There: Diaspora Policies, Integration, and Social Rights beyond Borders*, vol. 1. New York: Oxford University Press.

Desmond, Matthew, and Adam Travis. 2018. "Political Consequences of Survival Strategies among the Urban Poor." *American Sociological Review* 83(5, October): 869–96. DOI: https://doi.org/10.1177/0003122418792836.

De Souza Briggs, Xavier, Susan J. Popkin, and John Goering. 2010. *Moving to Opportunity: The Story of an American Experiment to Fight Ghetto Poverty.* Oxford: Oxford University Press.

Dill, Bonnie Thornton, Maxine Baca Zinn, and Sandra Patton. 1999. "Race, Family Values, and Welfare Reform." In *A New Introduction to Poverty: The Role of Race, Power, and Politics*, edited by Louis Kushnick and James Jennings. New York: New York University Press.

Dodd, S. J., and Jama Shelton. 2021. "Combatting Cisnormativity in Social Work Education, Research, and Practice." In *The Routledge International Handbook of Social Work and Sexualities*, edited by S. J. Dodd. London: Routledge.

Doussard, Marc. 2013. *Degraded Work: The Struggle at the Bottom of the Labor Market.* Minneapolis: University of Minnesota Press.

Dreby, Joanna. 2019. *Everyday Illegal: When Policies Undermine Immigrant Families.* Berkeley: University of California Press.

Dunbar-Ortiz, Roxanne. 2014. *An Indigenous Peoples' History of the United States.* Boston: Beacon Press.

Edin, Kathryn, and Laura Lein. 1997. *Making Ends Meet: How Single Mothers Survive Welfare and Low-Wage Work*. New York: Russell Sage Foundation.

Esping-Andersen, Gøsta, ed. 2002. *Why We Need a New Welfare State*. New York: Oxford University Press.

Faber, Jacob W. 2020. "We Built This: Consequences of New Deal Era Intervention in America's Racial Geography." *American Sociological Review* 85(5, October): 739–75. DOI: https://doi.org/10.1177/0003122420948464.

Fairbanks, Jesse. 2022. "Cities Experiment with Restitutive Housing Programs. Do They Advance Reparations?" Center for Law and Policy, February 28. https://www.clasp.org/blog/cities-experiment-restitutive-housing-programs-do-they-advance-reparations/.

Finch, Naomi. 2021. "Inclusive Citizenship and Degenderization: A Comparison of State Support in 22 European Countries." *Social Policy and Administration* 55(7, December): 1224–43. DOI: https://doi.org/10.1111/spol.12716.

Fine, Janice. 2006. *Worker Centers: Organizing Communities at the Edge of the Dream*. Ithaca, N.Y.: ILR Press.

Finney, Michael, and Renee Koury. 2021. "Bay Area Mom Waits 6 Months to Get EDD Benefits, Thousands More in Same Situation." *ABC-7 News*, November 10. https://abc7news.com/unemployment-edd-direct-deposit-ca-claims/11220888/.

Fix, Michael E., ed. 2009. *Immigrants and Welfare: The Impact of Welfare Reform on America's Newcomers*. New York: Russell Sage Foundation.

Fix, Michael, and Jeffrey Passel. 2002. "The Scope and Impact of Welfare Reform's Immigrant Provisions." Urban Institute, January. https://www.urban.org/sites/default/files/publication/60346/410412-Scope-and-Impact-of-Welfare-Reform-s-Immigrant-Provisions-The.PDF.

Fleming, Crystal M., Michèle Lamont, and Jessica S. Welburn. 2012. "African Americans Respond to Stigmatization: The Meanings and Salience of Confronting, Deflecting Conflict, Educating the Ignorant, and 'Managing the Self.'" *Ethnic and Racial Studies* 35(3): 400–417. DOI: https://doi.org/10.1080/01419870.2011.589527.

Fleming, Paul J., Laura Villa-Torres, Arianna Taboada, Chelly Richards, and Clare Barrington. 2017. "Marginalisation, Discrimination, and the Health of Latino Immigrant Day Labourers in a Central North Carolina Community." *Health and Social Care in the Community* 25(2, March): 527–37. DOI: https://doi.org/10.1111/hsc.12338.

Fox, Cybelle. 2012. *Three Worlds of Relief: Race, Immigration, and the American Welfare State from the Progressive Era to the New Deal*. Princeton, N.J.: Princeton University Press.

———. 2016. "Unauthorized Welfare: The Origins of Immigrant Status Restrictions in American Social Policy." *Journal of American History* 102(4, March): 1051–74. DOI: https://doi.org/10.1093/jahist/jav758.

———. 2019. "'The Line Must Be Drawn Somewhere': The Rise of Legal Status Restrictions in State Welfare Policy in the 1970s." *Studies in American Political Development* 33(2, October): 275–304. DOI: https://doi.org/10.1017/S0898588X19000129.

Galdas, Paul M., Francine Cheater, and Paul Marshall. 2005. "Men and Health Help-Seeking Behaviour: Literature Review." *Journal of Advanced Nursing* 49(6, March): 616–23. DOI: https://doi.org/10.1111/j.1365-2648.2004.03331.x.

Gallo, Sarah. 2016. "Humor in Father-Daughter Immigration Narratives of Resistance." *Anthropology and Education Quarterly* 47(3, September): 279–96. DOI: https://doi.org/10.1111/aeq.12156.

García, Angela S. 2020. "Undocumented, Not Unengaged: Local Immigration Laws and the Shaping of Undocumented Mexicans' Political Engagement." *Social Forces* 99(4, June): 1658–81. DOI: https://doi.org/10.1093/sf/soaa070.

García, Angela S., and Leah Schmalzbauer. 2017. "Placing Assimilation Theory: Mexican Immigrants in Urban and Rural America." *Annals of the American Academy of Political and Social Science* 672(1, July): 64–82. DOI: https://doi.org/10.1177/0002716217708565.

García Hernández, César Cuauhtémoc. 2014. "Creating Crimmigration." *Brigham Young University Law Review* 2013(6, February 28): 1457. https://digitalcommons.law.byu.edu/lawreview/vol2013/iss6/4.

Garip, Filiz. 2012. "Discovering Diverse Mechanisms of Migration: The Mexico–US Stream 1970–2000." *Population and Development Review* 38(3): 393–433. DOI: https://doi.org/10.1111/j.1728-4457.2012.00510.x.

Gast, Melanie Jones, and Dina G. Okamoto. 2016. "Moral or Civic Ties? Deservingness and Engagement among Undocumented Latinas in Non-profit Organisations." *Journal of Ethnic and Migration Studies* 42(12): 2013–30.

Gee, Lisa Christensen, Matthew Gardner, Misha E. Hill, and Meg Wiehe. 2017. "Undocumented Immigrants' State and Local Tax Contributions." Institute on Taxation and Economic Policy, March. https://itep.sfo2.digitaloceanspaces.com/immigration2017.pdf.

Gehi, Pooja. 2012. "Gendered (In)security: Migration and Criminalization in the Security State." *Harvard Journal of Law and Gender* 35(2): 357–98.

Geva, Dorit. 2011. "Not Just Maternalism: Marriage and Fatherhood in American Welfare Policy." *Social Politics: International Studies in Gender, State & Society* 18(1): 24–51. DOI: https://doi.org/10.1093/sp/jxr003.

Gleeson, Shannon. 2010. "Labor Rights for All? The Role of Undocumented Immigrant Status for Worker Claims Making." *Law and Social Inquiry* 35(3, Summer): 561–602. DOI: https://doi.org/10.1111/j.1747-4469.2010.01196.x.

Goffman, Alice. 2009. "On the Run: Wanted Men in a Philadelphia Ghetto." *American Sociology Review* 74(3, June): 339–57. DOI: https://doi.org/10.1177/000312240907400301.

Golash-Boza, Tanya, and Pierrette Hondagneu-Sotelo. 2013. "Latino Immigrant Men and the Deportation Crisis: A Gendered Racial Removal Program." *Latino Studies* 11(3): 271–92. DOI: https://doi.org/10.1057/lst.2013.14.

Goldman, Dana P., James P. Smith, and Nerraj Sood. 2005. "Legal Status and Health Insurance among Immigrants." *Health Affairs (Millwood)* 24(6, November/December): 1640–53. DOI: https://doi.org/10.1377/hlthaff.24.6.1640.

Griffith, Kati L. 2015. "Worker Centers and Labor Law Protections: Why Aren't They Having Their Cake?" *Berkeley Journal of Employment and Labor Law* 36(2): 331–49.

Hadley, Jack. 2003. "Sicker and Poorer—The Consequences of Being Uninsured: A Review of the Research on the Relationship between Health Insurance, Medical Care Use, Health, Work, and Income." *Medical Care Research and Review* 60(2, suppl., June): 3S–76S. DOI: https://doi.org/10.1177/1077558703254101.

Hamer, Jennifer, and Kathleen Marchioro. 2002. "Becoming Custodial Dads: Exploring Parenting among Low-Income and Working-Class African American Fathers." *Journal of Marriage and Family* 64(1): 116–29. DOI: https://doi.org/10.1111/j.1741-3737.2002.00116.x.

Hansen, Eric, and Martin Donohoe. 2003. "Health Issues of Migrant and Seasonal Farmworkers." *Journal of Health Care for the Poor and Underserved* 14(2, May): 153–64. DOI: https://doi.org/10.1353/hpu.2010.0790.

Harding, David J., Jessica J. B. Wyse, Cheyney Dobson, and Jeffrey D. Morenoff. 2014. "Making Ends Meet after Prison." *Journal of Policy Analysis and Management* 33(2, Spring): 440–70. DOI: https://doi.org/10.1002/pam.21741.

Hasdell, Rebecca. 2020. "What We Know about Basic Universal Income: A Cross-Synthesis of Reviews." Stanford Basic Income Lab, July. https://basicincome.stanford.edu/uploads/Umbrella%20Review%20BI_final.pdf.

Hayes, Joseph, and Laura Hill. 2017. "Undocumented Immigrants in California." Public Policy Institute of California, March. https://www.ppic.org/publication/undocumented-immigrants-in-california/ (accessed June 26, 2020).

Haynes, Chris, Jennifer L. Merolla, and S. Karthick Ramakrishnan. 2016. "Comprehensive Immigration Reform." In *Framing Immigrants: News Coverage, Public Opinion, and Policy*, edited by Chris Haynes, Jennifer L. Merolla, and S. Karthick Ramakrishnan. New York: Russell Sage Foundation.

Health Access. 2015. "Access to Care for Undocumented Californians by County (2015)." https://health-access.org/images/CountyMapOctober2015Revised.pdf.

Health Program of Alameda County (HealthPAC). 2018. "Participant Handbook." July. https://www.acgov.org/health/documents/HPACHandbook-en.pdf.

Healthy Alameda County. 2022. "Economy/Income, 2015–2019." Conduent Healthy Communities Institute. https://www.healthyalamedacounty.org/index.php?module=indicators&controller=index&action=indicatorsearch&doSearch=1&i=&l=238_132167_5597_5598_5599_5601_5602_5603_5604_5605_5606_5607_5608_5609_5613_5614_5616_5629_5630&t%5B%5D=38&primaryTopicOnly=&subgrouping=2&card=0&handpicked=0&resultsPerPage=150&showComparisons=1&showOnlySelectedComparisons=&showOnlySelectedComparisons=1&grouping=1&ordering=1&sortcomp=0&sortcompInclude Missing= (accessed May 27, 2022).

Henderson, Timothy J. 2011. *Beyond Borders: A History of Mexican Migration to the United States*. West Sussex, U.K.: Wiley-Blackwell.

Henderson, Debra, and Ann Tickamyer. 2009. "The Intersection of Poverty Discourses: Race, Class, Culture, and Gender." In *Emerging Intersections: Race, Class, and Gender in Theory, Policy, and Practice*, edited by Bonnie Thornton Dill and Ruth Enid Zambrana. New Brunswick, N.J.: Rutgers University Press.

Hennessy-Fiske, Molly. 2015. "Advocates Protest Latina Immigrant's Arrest at Texas Doctor's Office." *Los Angeles Times*, September 15.

Herd, Pamela, and Donald P. Moynihan. 2019. *Administrative Burden: Policymaking by Other Means*. New York: Russell Sage Foundation.

Hohle, Randolph. 2017. *Racism in the Neoliberal Era: A Meta History of Elite White Power*. New York: Routledge.

Holmes, Seth. 2013. *Fresh Fruit, Broken Bodies: Migrant Farmworkers in the United States*. Berkeley: University of California Press.

Immigrant Legal Resource Center. 2022. "Immigrant Families and the California Earned Income Tax Credit (CalEITC)." February. https://www.ilrc.org/sites/default/files/resources/ilrc_cal_eitc_february_2022.pdf.

Joassart-Marcelli, Pascale. 2013. "Ethnic Concentration and Nonprofit Organizations: The Political and Urban Geography of Immigrant Services in Boston, Massachusetts." *International Migration Review* 47(3, September): 730–72. DOI: https://doi.org/10.1111/imre.12041.

Johnson, Dawn Marie. 2001. "AEDPA and the IIRIRA: Treating Misdemeanors as Felonies for Immigration Purposes." *Journal of Legislation* 27(2): 477–91. https://scholarship.law.nd.edu/cgi/viewcontent.cgi?article=1161&context=jleg.

Jones-Correa, Michael. 1998. "Different Paths: Gender, Immigration, and Political Participation." *International Migration Review* 32(2, June): 326–49. https://doi.org /10.1177/019791839803200202.

Kaiser Family Foundation. 2023. "Health Coverage of Immigrants." December 20, 2022; updated March 30, 2023. https://www.kff.org/racial-equity-and-health -policy/fact-sheet/health-coverage-of-immigrants/#:~:text=Noncitizens%20are %20significantly%20more%20likely,in%20ten%20(8%25)%20citizens.

Katznelson, Ira. 2005. *When Affirmative Action Was White: An Untold History of Racial Inequality in Twentieth-Century America.* New York: W. W. Norton and Co.

Kaushal, Neeraj, and Robert Kaestner. 2005. "Welfare Reform and Health Insurance of Immigrants." *Health Services Research* 40(3, June): 697–721. DOI: https:// doi.org/10.1111/j.1475-6773.2005.00381.x.

Keliiaa, Caitlin. 2021. "Unsettling Domesticity: Native Women and U.S. Indian Policy in the San Francisco Bay Area." In Anti-Eviction Mapping Project, *Counterpoints: A San Francisco Bay Area Atlas of Displacement and Resistance.* New York: PM Press.

Kneebone, Elizabeth, and Alan Berube. 2014a. *Confronting Suburban Poverty in America.* Washington, D.C.: Brookings Institution Press.

———. 2014b. "Poverty and the Suburbs: An Introduction." In Kneebone and Berube, *Confronting Suburban Poverty in America.* Washington, D.C.: Brookings Institution Press.

Koech, Jasmine M., Jules P. Sostre, Gabriel M. Lockett, Kirsten A. Gonzalez, and Roberto L. Abreu. 2022. "Resisting by Existing: Trans Latinx Mental Health, Well-being, and Resilience in the United States." In *Latinx Queer Psychology*, edited by Reynel Alexander Chaparro and Marco Aurélio Máximo Prado. Switzerland: Springer Cham.

Kornbluh, Felicia, and Gwendolyn Mink. 2019. *Ensuring Poverty: Welfare Reform in Feminist Perspective.* Philadelphia: University of Pennsylvania Press.

KQED. 2017. *American Suburb* (podcast). NPR, September 20–22. https://www .npr.org/podcasts/552484922/american-suburb (accessed July 8, 2020).

Kulish, Nicholas. 2018. "What It Costs to Be Smuggled across the U.S. Border." *New York Times*, June 30.

Lamont, Michèle. 2000. *The Dignity of Working Men: Morality and the Boundaries of Race, Class, and Immigration.* Cambridge, Mass.: Harvard University Press.

Leff, Mark H. 1973. "Consensus for Reform: The Mothers' Pension Movement in the Progressive Era." *Social Service Review* 47(3): 397–417. DOI: https://doi.org /10.1086/643020.

Lei, Serena. 2015. "Nine Charts about Wealth Inequality in America (Updated)." Urban Institute, February 2015, updated October 24, 2017. https://apps.urban .org/features/wealth-inequality-charts/.

Leogrande, William M. 1990. "From Reagan to Bush: The Transition in U.S. Policy towards Central America." *Journal of Latin American Studies* 22(3, October): 595–621. DOI: https://doi.org/10.1017/S0022216X00020976.

Lichter, Daniel T., and Martha L. Crowley. 2004. "Welfare Reform and Child Poverty: Effects of Maternal Employment, Marriage, and Cohabitation." *Social Science Research* 33(3, September): 385–408. DOI: https://doi.org/10.1016/j.ssresearch .2003.09.001.

Lindsay, Brendan C. 2012. *Murder State: California's Native American Genocide, 1846–1873.* Lincoln: University of Nebraska Press.

Lohan, Maria. 2007. "How Might We Understand Men's Health Better? Integrating Explanations from Critical Studies on Men and Inequalities in Health." *Social Science and Medicine* 65(3, August): 493–504. DOI: https://doi.org/10.1016 /j.socscimed.2007.04.020.

Long, Peter. 2002. "Local Efforts to Increase Health Insurance Coverage among Children in California." Medi-Cal Policy Institute, February. https://www.chcf .org/wp-content/uploads/2017/12/PDF-LocalEffortsToInsureChildren.pdf.

Louie, Naomi T., Loan Pham Kim, and Scott E. Chan. 2020. "Perceptions and Barriers to SNAP Utilization among Asian and Pacific Islanders in Greater Los Angeles." *American Journal of Health Promotion* 34(7, September): 779–90. DOI: https:// doi.org/10.1177/0890117120925746.

Lowrey, Annie. 2021. "The Time Tax: Why Is So Much American Bureaucracy Left to Average Citizens?" *Atlantic*, July 27. https://www.theatlantic.com/politics /archive/2021/07/how-government-learned-waste-your-time-tax/619568/.

Loyd, Jenna, and Alison Mountz. 2018. *Boats, Borders, and Bases: Race, the Cold War, and the Rise of Migration Detention in the United States.* Berkeley: University of California Press.

Marrow, Helen. 2009. "Immigrant Bureaucratic Incorporation: The Dual Roles of Professional Missions and Government Policies." *American Sociological Review* 74(5, October):756–76. DOI: https://doi.org/10.1177/000312240907400504.

Massey, Douglas S. 1999. "Why Does Immigration Occur? A Theoretical Synthesis." In *The Handbook of International Migration: The American Experience*, edited by Charles Hirschman, Philip Kasinitz, and Josh DeWind. New York: Russell Sage Foundation.

Mayorkas, (Secretary) Alejandro N. 2021. "Guidelines for Enforcement Actions in or Near Protected Areas." Memo to ICE and USCIS directors, CBP commissioner, and officers of strategy, policy and plans, privacy, and civil rights and civil liberties. U.S. Department of Homeland Security, October 27. https://www.dhs.gov/sites /default/files/publications/21_1027_opa_guidelines-enforcement-actions-in-near -protected-areas.pdf (accessed January 22, 2022).

Médecins Sans Frontiers (Doctors Without Borders). 2017. "Forced to Flee Central America's Northern Triangle: A Neglected Humanitarian Crisis." May. https:// doctorswithoutborders.org/sites/default/files/2018-08/msf_forced-to-flee-central -americas-northern-triangle_E.pdf.

Menjívar, Cecilia. 2000. *Fragmented Ties: Salvadoran Immigrant Networks in America*. Berkeley: University of California Press.

Menjívar, Cecilia, and Leisy J. Abrego. 2012. "Legal Violence: Immigration Law and the Lives of Central American Immigrants." *American Journal of Sociology* 117(5, March): 1380–1421. DOI: https://doi.org/10.1086/663575.

Menjívar, Cecilia, Leisy J. Abrego, and Leah C. Schmalzbauer. 2016. *Immigrant Families*. Cambridge: Polity Press.

Minton, Sarah, and Linda Giannarelli. 2019. "Five Things You May Not Know about the U.S. Safety Net." Urban Institute, February. https://www.urban.org/sites /default/files/publication/99674/five_things_you_may_not_know_about_the_us _social_safety_net_1.pdf.

Molina, Natalia. 2006. *Fit to Be Citizens? Public Health and Race in Los Angeles, 1879–1939*. Berkeley: University of California Press.

———. 2011. "Borders, Laborers, and Racialized Medicalization." *American Journal of Public Health* 101(6, June): 1024–31. DOI: https://doi.org/10.2105/AJPH .2010.300056.

Monforton, Celeste, and Jane M. Von Bergen. 2021. *On the Job: The Untold Story of Worker Centers and the New Fight for Wages, Dignity, and Health*. New York: New Press.

Moskowitz, Peter E. 2017. *How to Kill a City: Gentrification, Inequality, and the Fight for the Neighborhood*. New York: Nation Books.

Moynihan, Donald, Pamela Herd, and Hope Harvey. 2014. "Administrative Burden: Learning, Psychological, and Compliance Costs in Citizen-State Interactions." *Journal of Public Administration Research and Theory* 25(1, January): 43–69. https:// doi.org/10.1093/jopart/muu009.

Mujeres Unidas y Activas, Day Labor Program Women's Collective of La Raza Centro Legal, and DataCenter. 2007. "Behind Closed Doors: Working Conditions of California Household Workers." DataCenter, March. http://www.datacenter.org /wp-content/uploads/behindcloseddoors.pdf.

Muñoz, Susana María, and Marta María Maldonado. 2012. "Counterstories of College Persistence by Undocumented Mexicana Students: Navigating Race, Class,

Gender, and Legal Status." *International Journal of Qualitative Studies in Education* 25(3, February 4): 293–315. DOI: https://doi.org/10.1080/09518398.2010 .529850.

Murphy, Alexandra K. 2010. "The Symbolic Dilemmas of Suburban Poverty: Challenges and Opportunities Posed by Variations in the Contours of Suburban Poverty." *Sociological Forum* 25(3, September): 541–69. DOI: https://doi.org /10.1111/j.1573-7861.2010.01195.x.

Murphy, Alexandra, and Danielle Wallace. 2010. "Opportunities for Making Ends Meet and Upward Mobility: Differences in Organizational Deprivation across Urban and Suburban Poor Neighborhoods." *Social Science Quarterly* 91(5, December): 1164–86. DOI: https://doi.org/10.1111/j.1540-6237.2010.00726.x.

Myers, Ana McCormick, and Matthew A. Painter. 2017. "Food Insecurity in the United States of America: An Examination of Race/Ethnicity and Nativity." *Food Security* 9(November 22): 1419–32. DOI: https://doi.org/10.1007/s12571 -017-0733-8.

Myles, John, and Jill Quadagno. 2002. "Political Theories of the Welfare State." *Social Service Review* 76(1, March): 34–57. DOI: https://doi.org/10.1086/324607.

Nadasen, Premilla. 2007. "From Widow to 'Welfare Queen': Welfare and the Politics of Race." *Black Women, Gender, and Families* 1(2, Fall): 52–77.

Nadeem, Erum, Jane M. Lange, Dawn Edge, Maria Fongwa, Tom Belin, and Jeanne Miranda. 2007. "Does Stigma Keep Poor Young Immigrant and U.S.-Born Black and Latina Women from Seeking Mental Health Care?" *Psychiatry Services* 58(12): 1547–54. DOI: https://doi.org/10.1176/appi.ps.58.12.1547.

National Immigration Law Center. 2017. "New Evidence Proves Deported DACA Recipient Juan Manuel Montes Was Kicked Out of the U.S. by Immigration Officials against His Will." July 14. https://www.nilc.org/2017/07/14/new-evidence -proves-deported-daca-recipient-juan-manuel-montes-was-kicked-out-of-the-u -s-by-immigration-officials-against-his-will/ (accessed August 29, 2017).

Neuberger, Zoë, and Robert Greenstein. 2004. "WIC-Only Stores and Competitive Pricing in the WIC Program." Center on Budget and Policy Priorities, May 17. https://www.cbpp.org/sites/default/files/atoms/files/5-17-04wic.pdf.

Newfield, Chris. 2011. *Unmaking the Public University: The Forty-Year Assault on the Middle Class.* Cambridge, Mass.: Harvard University Press.

Nicholls, Walter J., Marcel Maussen, and Laura Caldas de Mesquita. 2016. "The Politics of Deservingness." *American Behavioral Scientist* 60(13, November): 1590–1612. DOI: https://doi.org/10.1177/0002764216664944.

Ngai, Mae M. 2014. *Impossible Subjects: Illegal Aliens and the Making of Modern America.* Princeton, N.J.: Princeton University Press.

O'Connor, Allison, Jeanne Batalova, and Jessica Bolter. 2019. "Central American Immigrants in the United States." Migration Policy Institute, August 15. https://www.migrationpolicy.org/article/central-american-immigrants-united-states-2017.

Office of Governor Gavin Newsom. 2022. "California Expands Medi-Cal to All Eligible Adults 50 Years of Age and Older." April 29. https://www.gov.ca.gov/2022/04/29/california-expands-medi-cal-to-all-eligible-adults-50-years-of-age-and-older/ (accessed May 28, 2022).

Opillard, Florian. 2015. "Resisting the Politics of Displacement in the San Francisco Bay Area: Anti-Gentrification Activism in the Tech Boom 2.0." *European Journal of American Studies* 10(3). DOI: https://doi.org/10.4000/ejas.11322.

Organization for Economic Cooperation and Development (OECD). 2019. "Inequalities." In *Society at a Glance: OECD Social Indicators: A Spotlight on LGBT People.* Paris: OECD Publishing. DOI: https://doi.org/10.1787/19991290.

Orloff, Ann Shola. 1993. *The Politics of Pensions: A Comparative Analysis of Britain, Canada, and the United States, 1880–1940.* Madison: University of Wisconsin Press.

Orloff, Ann Shola, and Theda Skocpol. 1984. "Why Not Equal Protection? Explaining the Politics of Public Social Spending in Britain, 1900–1911, and the United States, 1880s–1920." *American Sociological Review* 49(6, December): 726–50. DOI: https://doi.org/10.2307/2095527.

Osorio, Liliana, Hilda Dávila, and Xóchitl Castañeda. 2019. "Binational Health Week: A Social Mobilization Program to Improve Latino Migrant Health." In *Accountability across Borders: Migrant Rights in North America*, edited by Xóchitl Bada and Shannon Gleeson. Austin: University of Texas Press.

O'Toole, Molly. 2020. "Trump Defies Supreme Court by Denying New DACA Applications." *Los Angeles Times*, July 16.

Palomino, Joaquin. 2015. "As Bay Area Poverty Shifts from Cities to Suburbia, Services Lag." *San Francisco Chronicle*, December 31. Updated January 2, 2016. https://www.sfchronicle.com/bayarea/article/As-poverty-spreads-to-new-Bay-Area-suburbs-6730818.php (accessed July 15, 2020).

Panchok-Berry, Andrea, Alex R. Rivas, and Alexandra K. Murphy. 2013. "Shifting Settlement Patterns and Mismatched Resources: The Landscape of Immigrant Organizations in Urban and Suburban Philadelphia." *SSRN Electronic Journal* (January). DOI: https://doi.org/10.2139/ssrn.2318088.

Park, Lisa Sun-Hee. 2011. *Entitled to Nothing: The Struggle for Immigrant Health Care in the Age of Welfare Reform.* New York: New York University, Press.

Perreira, Krista M., and India Ornelas. 2013. "Painful Passages: Traumatic Experiences and Post-Traumatic Stress among Immigrant Latino Adolescents and Their Primary

Caregivers." *International Migration Review* 47(4, December): 976–1005. DOI: https://doi.org/10.1111/imre.12050.

Philadelphia Inquirer. 2021. "A New Kind of Union Emerges for Lower Paid Workers across the U.S." *Philadelphia Inquirer*, May 29. https://www.inquirer.com/business/worker-center-jobs-labor-union-rights-poultry-farm-poor-20210529.html.

Prieto, Greg. 2018. *Immigrants under Threat: Risk and Resistance in Deportation Nation.* New York: New York University Press.

Rank, Mark R. 2010. "Poverty and Its Effects." In *Mental Health and Social Problems*, edited by Nina Rovinelli Heller and Alex Gitterman. London: Routledge.

Rasmussen, Andrew, Barry Rosenfeld, Kim Reeves, and Allen S. Keller. 2007. "The Subjective Experience of Trauma and Subsequent PTSD in a Sample of Undocumented Immigrants." *Journal of Nervous and Mental Disease* 195(2, February): 137–43. DOI: https://doi.org/10.1097/01.nmd.0000254748.38784.2f.

Reese, Ellen. 2011. *They Say Cut Back, We Say Fight Back! Welfare Activism in an Era of Retrenchment.* New York: Russell Sage Foundation.

Ro, Annie, Jennifer Van Hook, and Katrina M. Walsemann. 2022. "Undocumented Older Latino Immigrants in the United States: Population Projections and Share of Older Undocumented Latinos by Health Insurance Coverage and Chronic Health Conditions, 2018–2038." *Journals of Gerontology: Series B, Psychological Sciences and Social Sciences* 77(2, February 3): 389–95. DOI: https://doi.org/10.1093/geronb/gbab189.

Romani, Maria. 2022. "Collusion in California's Central Valley: The Case for Ending Sheriff Entanglement with ICE." American Civil Liberties Union of Northern California, February. https://www.aclunc.org/sites/default/files/ICE_report_10_2-11-22-final-web.pdf.

Rook, Karen S., Kristin J. August, Mary Ann Parris Stephens, and Melissa M. Franks. 2011. "When Does Spousal Social Control Provoke Negative Reactions in the Context of Chronic Illness? The Pivotal Role of Patients' Expectations." *Journal of Social and Personal Relationships* 28(6, September). DOI: https://doi.org/10.1177/0265407510391335.

Rosales, Rocío. 2020. *Fruteros: Street Vending, Illegality, and Ethnic Community in Los Angeles.* Berkeley: University of California Press.

Ross, Janelle. 2016. "From Mexican Rapists to Bad Hombres, the Trump Campaign in Two Moments." *Washington Post*, October 20. https://www.washingtonpost.com/news/the-fix/wp/2016/10/20/from-mexican-rapists-to-bad-hombres-the-trump-campaign-in-two-moments/.

Roth, Benjamin J., and Scott W. Allard. 2016. "(Re)Defining Access to Latino Immigrant-Serving Organizations: Evidence from Los Angeles, Chicago, and Washington, D.C." *Journal of the Society for Social Work and Research* 7(4, Winter): 729–53. DOI: https://doi.org/10.1086/689358.

Saxonberg, Steven. 2013. "From Defamilialization to Degenderization: Toward a New Welfare Typology." *Social Policy and Administration* 47(1, February): 26–49. DOI: https://doi.org/10.1111/j.1467-9515.2012.00836.x.

Schafran, Alex. 2019. *The Road to Resegregation: Northern California and the Failure of Politics*. Berkeley: University of California Press.

Schanzenbach, Diane, and Natalie Tomeh. 2020. "Visualizing Food Insecurity." Institute for Policy Research, July 14. https://www.ipr.northwestern.edu/state-food-insecurity.html (accessed December 5, 2021).

Schmalzbauer, Leah. 2014. *The Last Best Place? Gender, Family, and Migration in the New West*. Redwood City, Calif.: Stanford University Press.

Schram, Sanford F., Joe Soss, Richard C. Fording, and Linda Houser. 2009. "Deciding to Discipline: Race, Choice, and Punishment at the Frontlines of Welfare Reform." *American Sociological Review* 74(3, June): 398–422. DOI: https://doi.org/10.1177/000312240907400304.

Scott, James C. 1985. *Weapons of the Weak: Everyday Forms of Peasant Resistance*. New Haven, Conn.: Yale University Press.

———. 1990. *Hidden Transcripts: Domination and the Arts of Resistance*. New Haven, Conn.: Yale University Press.

Seif, Hinda. 2014. "'Layers of Humanity': Interview with Undocuqueer Artivist Julio Salgado." *Latino Studies* 12(2): 300–309. DOI: https://doi.org/10.1057/lst.2014.31.

———. 2016. "'Coming Out of the Shadows' and 'Undocuqueer': Undocumented Immigrants Transforming Sexuality Discourse and Activism." In *Queering Borders: Language, Sexuality, and Migration*, vol. 85, edited by D.A.B. Murray. Amsterdam: John Benjamins Publishing Co.

Singer, Audrey, Susan W. Hardwick, and Caroline B. Bretell, eds. 2008. *Twenty-First Century Gateways: Immigrant Incorporation in Suburban America*. Washington, D.C.: Brookings Institution Press.

Skocpol, Theda. 1992. *Protecting Soldiers and Mothers: The Political Origins of Social Policy in the United States*. Cambridge, Mass.: Belknap Press of Harvard University Press.

Slack, Jeremy, and Daniel E. Martínez. 2018. "What Makes a Good Human Smuggler? The Differences between Satisfaction with and Recommendation of Coyotes on the

U.S.-Mexico Border." *Annals of the American Academy of Political and Social Science* 676(1, March): 152–73. DOI: https://doi.org/10.1177/0002716217750562.

Small, Mario Luis. 2009. *Unanticipated Gains: Origins of Network Inequality in Everyday Life.* Oxford: Oxford University Press.

Sosa, Anabel. 2022. "A Historic Achievement: California Expands Medi-Cal to All Low-Income Residents." UC Berkeley Labor Center, November 7. https://laborcenter.berkeley.edu/a-historic-achievement/.

Soss, Joe Brian. 2000a. *Unwanted Claims: The Politics of Participation in the U.S. Welfare System.* Ann Arbor: University of Michigan Press.

———. 2000b. "Welfare Claiming as Survival Politics." In Soss, *Unwanted Claims: The Politics of Participation in the U.S. Welfare System.* Ann Arbor: University of Michigan Press.

Soss, Joe, Richard C. Fording, and Sanford F. Schram. 2011. *Disciplining the Poor: Neoliberal Paternalism and the Persistent Power of Race.* Chicago: University of Chicago Press.

Stack, Carol B. 1974. *All Our Kin: Strategies for Survival in a Black Community.* New York: Harper & Row.

Stern, Alexandra M. 2005. *Eugenic Nation: Faults and Frontiers of Better Breeding in Modern America.* Berkeley: University of California Press.

Stumpf, Juliet. 2006. "The Crimmigration Crisis: Immigrants, Crime, and Sovereign Power." *American University Law Review* 56(2, December): 367–419.

Stutzer, Alois, and Bruno S. Frey. 2008. "Stress That Doesn't Pay: The Commuting Paradox." *Scandinavian Journal of Economics* 110(2, June): 339–66. DOI: https://doi.org/10.1111/j.1467-9442.2008.00542.x.

Suro, Roberto, and Hannah Findling. 2020. "State and Local Aid for Immigrants during the COVID-19 Pandemic: Innovating Inclusion." *Computational Management Science* (January). DOI: https://doi.org/10.14240/cmsesy070820.

Torres-Pinzon, Diana L., Walter Solorzano, Sue E. Kim, and Michael R. Cousineau. 2020. "Coronavirus Disease 2019 and the Case to Cover Undocumented Immigrants in California." *Health Equity* 4(1, November 25): 500–504. DOI: https://doi.org/10.1089/heq.2020.0049.

University of California–Los Angeles. 2022. "Undocumented UC Student Organizers, Professors from UCLA CILP, and Labor Center Launch Groundbreaking Campaign for Equal Access to Job Opportunities." Center for Immigration Law and Policy, October 19. https://www.labor.ucla.edu/press-release/undocumented-uc-student-organizers-professors-from-ucla-cilp-labor-center-launch-groundbreaking-campaign-for-equal-access-to-job-opportunities/.

U.S. Census Bureau. 2020a. "American Community Survey (ACS) 5-Year Estimates Subject Tables: Poverty Status in the past 12 months, Oakland City, California." https://data.census.gov/table?t=Income+and+Poverty&g=040XX00US06_160XX 00US0653000&y=2020&tid=ACSST5Y2020.S1701 (accessed September 2023).

———. 2020b. "American Community Survey (ACS) 5-Year Estimates Subject Tables: Poverty Status in the past 12 months, Concord City, California." https://data .census.gov/table?t=Income+and+Poverty&g=040XX00US06_160XX00US0616000 &y=2020&tid=ACSST5Y2020.S1701 (accessed September 2023).

———. 2020c. "American Community Survey (ACS) 5-Year Estimates Subject Tables: Poverty Status in the past 12 months, Antioch City, California." https://data.census .gov/table?t=Income+and+Poverty&g=040XX00US06_160XX00US0602252&y =2020&tid=ACSST5Y2020.S1701 (accessed September 2023).

———. 2020d. "American Community Survey (ACS) 5-Year Estimates Data Profiles, Demographic and Housing Estimates, Antioch City, California." https://data.census .gov/table?g=160XX00US0602252&y=2020&tid=ACSDP5Y2020.DP05 (accessed September 2023).

———. 2020e. "American Community Survey (ACS) 5-Year Estimates Data Profiles, Demographic and Housing Estimates, Concord City, California." https://data .census.gov/table?g=160XX00US0616000&y=2020&tid=ACSDP5Y2020.DP05 (accessed September 2023).

———. 2020f. "American Community Survey (ACS) 5-Year Estimates Data Profiles, Demographic and Housing Estimates, Oakland City, California." https:// data.census.gov/table?q=dp05&g=160XX00US0653000&y=2020 (accessed September 2023).

———. n.d.-a. "Antioch City, California Profile, 2021 ACS 5-Year Estimates Data Profiles." https://data.census.gov/profile/Antioch_city,_California?g =160XX00US0602252 (accessed September 2023)

———. n.d.-b. "Concord City, California Profile, 2021 ACS 5-Year Estimates Data Profiles." https://data.census.gov/profile/Concord_city,_California?g =160XX00US0616000 (accessed September 2023).

———. n.d.-c. "Oakland City, California Profile, 2021 ACS 5-Year Estimates Data Profiles." https://data.census.gov/profile/Oakland_city,_California?g =160XX00US0653000 (accessed September 2023).

———. n.d.-d. "Quick Facts: Alameda County, California." https://www.census.gov /quickfacts/alamedacountycalifornia (accessed May 27, 2022).

———. n.d.-e. "Quick Facts: Antioch City, California." https://www.census.gov /quickfacts/fact/table/antiochcitycalifornia/PST045221 (accessed May 27, 2022).

———. n.d.-f. "Quick Facts: Concord City, California." https://www.census .gov/quickfacts/fact/table/concordcitycalifornia/PST045221 (accessed May 27, 2022).

———. n.d.-g. "Quick Facts: Oakland City, California." https://www.census.gov /quickfacts/fact/table/oaklandcitycalifornia/PST045221 (accessed May 27, 2022).

U.S. Citizenship and Immigration Services. 2022. "Update on Ramos v. Nielsen." Updated November 14, 2022. https://www.uscis.gov/humanitarian/update-on -ramos-v-nielsen.

U.S. Department of Agriculture. 2019. "WIC 2016 Eligibility and Coverage Rates." Food and Nutrition Service. https://www.fns.usda.gov/wic/wic-2016-eligibility -and-coverage-rates.

U.S. Department of the Treasury. 2021. "FACT SHEET: The American Rescue Plan Will Deliver Immediate Economic Relief to Families." March 18. https://home .treasury.gov/news/featured-stories/fact-sheet-the-american-rescue-plan-will -deliver-immediate-economic-relief-to-families.

Valenzuela, Abel, Nik Theodore, Edwin Meléndez, and Ana Luz Gonzalez. 2006. "On the Corner: Day Labor in the United States." Center for the Study of Urban Poverty, January. https://www.issuelab.org/resources/478/478.pdf.

Van Hook, Jennifer, and Kelly Stamper Balistreri. 2006. "Ineligible Parents, Eligible Children: Food Stamps Receipt, Allotments, and Food Insecurity among Children of Immigrants." *Social Science Research* 35(1, March): 228–51. DOI: https://doi.org /10.1016/j.ssresearch.2004.09.001.

Vidal de Haymes, Maria, Siobhan O'Donoghue, and Hien Nguyen. 2019. "The Impact of School-Based Volunteering on Social Capital and Self- and Collective Efficacy among Low-Income Mothers." *Children and Schools* 41(2, April): 79–88. DOI: https://doi.org/10.1093/cs/cdz005.

Vidal-Ortiz, Salvador, and Juliana Martínez. 2018. "Latinx Thoughts: Latinidad with an X." *Latino Studies* 16(3): 384–95. DOI: https://doi.org/10.1057/s41276-018 -0137-8.

Villarejo, Don, and Stephen A. McCurdy. 2008. "The California Agricultural Workers Health Survey." *Journal of Agricultural Safety and Health* 14(2, April): 135–46. DOI: https://doi.org/10.13031/2013.24347.

Vogt, Wendy A. 2018. *Lives in Transit: Violence and Intimacy on the Migrant Journey.* Berkeley: University of California Press.

Vollinger, Ellen. 2022. "Federal Nutrition Programs Are among Gateways for Internet Service Discounts." Food Research and Action Center, May 12. https://frac.org /blog/affordable-connectivity-program.

Wakefield, Mary. 2021. "Federally Qualified Health Centers and Related Primary Care Workforce Issues." *Journal of the American Medical Association* 325(12): 1145–46. DOI: https://doi.org/10.1001/jama.2021.1964.

Walsemann, Katrina M., Annie Ro, and Gilbert C. Gee. 2017. "Trends in Food Insecurity among California Residents from 2001 to 2011: Inequities at the Intersection of Immigration Status and Ethnicity." *Preventive Medicine* 105(December): 142–48. DOI: https://doi.org/10.1016/j.ypmed.2017.09.007.

Webb Hooper, Monica, Anna María Nápoles, and Eliseo J. Pérez-Stable. 2020. "COVID-19 and Racial/Ethnic Disparities." *Journal of the American Medical Association* 323(24, June 23): 2466–67. DOI: https://doi.org/10.1001/jama.2020.8598.

Weil, David. 2014. *The Fissured Workplace: Why Work Became So Bad for So Many and What can Be Done to Improve It.* Cambridge, Mass.: Harvard University Press.

Weir, Margaret, Ann Shola Orloff, and Theda Skocpol. 1988. *The Politics of Social Policy in the United States*, vol. 2. Princeton, N.J.: Princeton University Press.

Weir, Margaret, Nancy Pindus, Howard Wial, and Harold Wolman. 2012. "Building a Resilient Social Safety Net." In *Urban and Regional Policy and Its Effects*, vol. 4, edited by Margaret Weir, Howard Wial, Harold Wolman, and Nancy Pindus. Washington, D.C.: Brookings Institution Press.

White House. 2021. "Executive Order on Advancing Racial Equity and Support for Underserved Communities through the Federal Government." White House Briefing Room, January 20. https://www.whitehouse.gov/briefing-room/presidential-actions/2021/01/20/executive-order-advancing-racial-equity-and-support-for-underserved-communities-through-the-federal-government/.

———. 2022. "Biden Administration Announces State-by-State Funding to Address Home Energy Costs." White House Briefing Room, January 7. https://www.whitehouse.gov/briefing-room/statements-releases/2022/01/07/biden-administration-announces-state-by-state-funding-to-address-home-energy-costs/.

Williams, David R. 2003. "The Health of Men: Structured Inequalities and Opportunities." *American Journal of Public Health* 93(5, May): 724–31. DOI: https://doi.org/10.2105/ajph.93.5.724.

Williams, David R., Jourdyn A. Lawrence, and Brigette A. Davis. 2019. "Racism and Health: Evidence and Needed Research." *Annual Review of Public Health* 40: 105–25. DOI: https://doi.org/10.1146/annurev-publhealth-040218-043750.

Wimmer, Andreas. 2008. "Elementary Strategies of Ethnic Boundary Making." *Ethnic and Racial Studies* 31(6): 1025–55. DOI: https://doi.org/10.1080/01419870801905612.

Wroe, Andrew. 2008. "The Judicial Death of Proposition 187." In Wroe, *The Republican Party and Immigration Politics: From Proposition 187 to George W. Bush.* New York: Palgrave Macmillan.

Yoshikawa, Hirokazu. 2011. *Immigrants Raising Citizens: Undocumented Parents and Their Young Children.* New York: Russell Sage Foundation.

Zhou, Min. 2009. "How Neighbourhoods Matter for Immigrant Children: The Formation of Educational Resources in Chinatown, Koreatown, and Pico Union, Los Angeles." *Journal of Ethnic and Migration Studies* 35(7): 1153–79. DOI: https://doi.org/10.1080/13691830903006168.

INDEX

Tables and figures are listed in **boldface**.

narrative frames: of DREAMer
movement, 119–20; effective,
in lobbying for immigration
reform, 121, 132–33. *See also*
counternarratives of immigrants in
response to stigmatization
nonprofit organizations (NPOs), social
service: in Antioch, **55**, 57; author's
work with, 146–47; in Concord, **55**,
57; and expansion of immigrants'
social capital, 84; legal aid NPOs,
50, 58–60, 69–70, 154n26; as less
common in suburbs, 67–68, 123;
in Oakland, **55**, 56; outreach to
immigrants, need for research on, 84

Oakland, California: author's work at
nonprofit organizations in, 13;
culturally specific care in, 57;
day labor organizations in, 42;
demographics, **55**, 56; demographics
of sample respondents, **15**, 19;
FQHCs in, 60–61; geography of,
54; legal aid NPO staffing, 59–60,
154n26; location of, **12**, 52, **53**;
median household income, 26, 56;
as one site for this study, 12; poverty
levels, 53, **54**, **55**; and primary care
access, 82; safety net infrastructure,
55, 56, 57; undocumented
immigrants' eligibility for
HealthPAC, 101

Pandemic EBT (P-EBT), 138
Personal Responsibility and Work
Opportunity Reconciliation Act of
1996 (PRWORA), 24–25, 152n8

police: abuse and discrimination by, 70;
collusion with ICE, 157n28; work to
build immigrants' trust, 69–70
policy implications of this research,
129–35
poverty: blaming people in, 6; impact
on mental health, 38–39; needed
adjustments to definition of, 134
prenatal services for immigrants: access
to other services through, 74, 76,
80–81; eligibility in California, **27**,
31–33, **32**; states requiring qualified
immigration status, 31
PRWORA. *See* Personal Responsibility
and Work Opportunity
Reconciliation Act of 1996
public charge rule, 137

race: and eligibility for government
programs, 7–8, 9, 23–24; and
structural violence, 39; in supervision
of benefit recipients, 8

safety net, U.S.: and administrative
burdens, 127; Biden administration
and, 139; conditional care in, 5, 123;
COVID-19 pandemic and, 139;
"crash pads" for those excluded from,
5, 72, 99–100; decreased spending
after 1950s, 7; and "deserving"
standard, replacement of, 134–35;
gender differences in access to, 125;
as historically exclusive, 2; history of,
7; impact of immigration status
and place on access to, 124–25;
improvement of, as best avenue for
immigration reform, 122; need for

welfare programs in U.S. *See* safety net, U.S.

WIC. *See* Special Supplemental Nutrition Program for Women, Infants, and Children

women: access to support network or guiding figure and, 18–19, 72, 77–79, 84–85, 90; greater interface with institutions than men, 10; and migration, 18; openness to interview process, 144; resistance to exploitation, 107

women's health, in undocumented immigrants: access to services through motherhood, 8, 10, 20–21, 31–33, 42–45, 90, 103; difficulty of finding primary care, 82–83; lack of health insurance, 93; limited access to health care, 93–95; and risks of seeking care, 74–76. *See also* gender; prenatal services for immigrants

work. *See* labor conditions for undocumented populations

worker centers/day labor centers: and immigration activism, 120; men connecting to health care through, 100, 101–3; men connecting to resources through, 101, 102–3; men connecting to work through, 100; need for greater number of, 130–31; services provided by, 46, 87, 90–91; as small bandage on structural violence of larger system, 103–4; variation in programs offered, 104

workers' compensation, undocumented workers and, 46, 94

working-class men, and moral boundaries, 119

work narrative of undocumented immigrants, 106, 110–13, 121

workplace injuries, uninsured immigrants and, 89